MEDICAL PHYSICISTS AND MALPRACTICE

MEDICAL PHYSICISTS AND MALPRACTICE

by

Robert J. Shalek, Ph.D., J.D.   *and*   **David S. Gooden, Ph.D., J.D.**
Professor Emeritus   Director
Department of Radiation Physics   *Department of Biomedical Physics*
The University of Texas   Saint Francis Hospital
M.D. Anderson Cancer Center   Tulsa, Oklahoma
Houston, Texas

Best wishes
Robert Shalek
July 24, 1996.

With regards —
David S. Gooden
July 1996

Medical Physics Publishing

———

Madison, Wisconsin

Library of Congress Cataloging-in-Publication Data

Shalek, Robert J.
    Medical physicists and malpractice / by Robert J. Shalek and David
S. Gooden.
        p.   cm.
    Includes bibliographical references and index.
    ISBN 0-944838-64-2 (hardcover). — ISBN 0-944838-65-0 (soft)
    1. Radiologists—Malpractice—United States. 2. Physical
therapists—Malpractice—United States. I. Gooden, David S. II. Title.
    KF2910.R333S53   1996
    346.7303'32—dc20
    [347.306332]
                                                          96-17117
                                                              CIP

Medical Physics Publishing
4513 Vernon Blvd.
Madison, WI 53705
608-262-4021

Design and Composition by Colophon Typesetting

Information given in this book is for instructional use only. The authors,
publisher, and printer take no responsibility for any damage or harm
incurred as a result of this information.

CONTENTS

CHAPTER 4 ⊞ THE LEGAL DUTY OF MEDICAL PHYSICISTS 37

CHAPTER 5 ⊞ REDUCING LIABILITY EXPOSURE — Reducing the Probability of Being Sued and Improving a Defense If Sued 47

CHAPTER 6 ⊞ SOME MALPRACTICE CASES INVOLVING MEDICAL PHYSICISTS 55

PREFACE

We both have primary careers in medical physics and attended law school in the evening while working as medical physicists. Law and medical physics are each demanding professions, and one person cannot pursue both simultaneously. However, we believe that our medical physics experience, our legal training, and our encounters with the legal system, particularly as expert witnesses, give us something useful to say to practicing medical physicists. While this book is written for medical physicists, nearly all of it will be useful to radiation oncologists and diagnostic radiologists. Dosimetrists and radiation therapists will also find this book of interest.

Another title for this book might have been, "Some Messages from the Courts to Medical Physicists." This is partly a how-to book about staying out of legal trouble, but we also intend for it to give insight into how society deals with injuries that a patient alleges were caused by health care professionals, institutions, or manufacturers of products. We briefly discuss pertinent theories of substantive law, civil legal procedure, and rules of evidence. Emphasis has been given to aspects of these subjects that will help keep a physicist out of court or improve a physicist's position in court. We include a list of quality assurance principles for physics related to radiation therapy, nuclear medicine, and diagnostic radiology. Some of these principles have been derived from malpractice cases. We discuss a number of incidents and malpractice cases involving physics in radiation oncology and give physics comments and legal comments. These cases are meant to exemplify various types of physics errors. Other incidents that have occurred are discussed briefly conveying just the nature and magnitude of the physics error.

Another chapter examines the origin of the legal duty of a medical physicist to a patient and looks at the responsibilities of medical physicists as elaborated in various American Association of Physicists in Medicine (AAPM) reports. This effort is more of a work in progress than a final statement. We hope that this discussion will be included in AAPM policy considerations.

Our hope is that medical physicists will read our book and conduct their business in a way that will reduce their exposure to liability while improving their professional performance. We have tried to indicate where we express opinions, but surely we have not succeeded completely in separating what we regard as fact from opinion. In chapter eight, "Editorial and Professional Views," we have indulged in opinion without restraint.

Medical professionals respond in different ways to becoming defendants in malpractice lawsuits. Some respond emotionally with suicide, disappearance, quitting practice, or returning to a training program. Others take the events in stride as part of the professional risk. We include a story called "A Medical Physicist Encounters the Law," told in four episodes throughout the book. In this story we have tried to convey some of the feelings of a defendant. More importantly, in describing some of the salient pretrial and trial steps, we hope to indicate that the many legal events are small steps that need not be overwhelming.

April 1996
RJS
DSG

ACKNOWLEDGMENTS

We have pursued two laudable goals that at times seemed contradictory —reasonable correctness and reader interest. To the extent that we have been successful in this pursuit we give acknowledgment and thanks to our strong-minded critics.

Ernest (Skip) Reynolds III is an honors graduate of the University of Texas School of Law and an experienced trial attorney in Fort Worth representing defendants. He gave generously of his time, corrected our sometimes overly theoretical law, and wrote or rewrote more than a few of the better passages.

John Cameron, a distinguished medical physicist, worked very conscientiously as an agent of the publisher on behalf of the reader asking for simplicity and clarity. Probably 90% of his suggestions are in the book.

Kimberly Herrick is an editorial consultant at M.D. Anderson. She worked over the manuscript carefully untangling syntax tangles.

Barbara Pylate is a continuing education specialist at M.D. Anderson. She typed and retyped the manuscript a number of times making logical and organizational recommendations along the way. Her ingenuity and simple assurance that it could be done were valuable. Her unflappable composure was much appreciated.

It appears that the Library of Congrss data is incorrect in some respects. When faced with the choice of delaying publication or publishing as is, we chose to meet our schedule.

PROLOGUE

§ 1 A Medical Physicist Encounters the Law (1)

As usual, Barbara Hickman, board certified in therapeutic radiological physics, enjoyed her 23-minute drive to the Mountain View Cancer Center. Today's early June sunrise was especially beautiful. Ms. Hickman was surprised to see a car in the parking lot. She usually beat everyone, including radiation oncologist Dr. Thomas Brewster, to the treatment center. Ms. Hickman parked in her usual spot several spaces to the right of a well-used 1988 Ford Fairlane. The young man in the driver's seat appeared unaccustomed to his white dress shirt and tie. He smiled courteously. Although Ms. Hickman did not recognize the man, she did not find him threatening. Smiling in his direction, she grabbed her purse and briefcase, opened the door, and stepped out of the car. Before she could close the door, the stranger, still smiling, was at her side. "Ms. Hickman?" he asked politely. Her lips were still in the process of forming "yes" when the young man produced an official looking envelope from his right hip pocket. His outstretched arm invited her to take the envelope. Pressing her purse to her side with her elbow, she offered fingers strung with car keys to accept it. The young man thrust the envelope into her hand. In what seemed a single action, he said, "Have a nice day!" got into his car, and drove away.

Confused by these strange events, Barbara Hickman stood motionless for some time. Then she became acutely aware of the envelope. She tossed the briefcase and purse on the car seat, placed the key ring between her teeth, and quickly opened the envelope. The document said in part:

"Defendant, Greetings: You are required to appear by filing a written answer to the enclosed plaintiff's petition at or before 10 o'clock A.M. of the Monday next after the expiration of 20 days after the date of service thereof in Blaire County District Court in the medical malpractice matter of *Marvin G. Stifler v. Thomas T. Brewster, M.D., Barbara M. Hickman, M.S., and Mountain View Cancer Center"*

Ms. Hickman read the words several times trying to understand their meaning. "My God," she thought, "I'm being sued."

For the next few years, the lawsuit will never be completely out of Barbara Hickman's mind. It will consume inordinate amounts of her time and energy. It will compromise her ability to perform at her peak professional capacity. It will strain her relationships with family and friends. It will dilute her personal and professional reputation. Ms. Hickman will not come out of this unaffected.

(This story is continued in § 16.)

1

BASIS OF THE LAW

§ 2 Introduction to Malpractice Law—Torts

A patient who believes that he or she has received improper medical treatment may be entitled to take legal action against those who administered that treatment. Typically, all persons, institutions, and organizational entities involved with the treatment are named as defendants. That is, everybody is sued. Physicists may be among the defendants named, especially if radiation dose or imaging quality is an issue. A medical physicist is most likely to be sued for negligence or, if the physicist sells products, possibly under a products liability theory. Both negligence and products liability are torts. A tort is difficult to define.

> Broadly speaking, a tort is a civil wrong, other than breach of contract, for which the court will provide a remedy in the form of an action for damages . . . . So far as there is one central idea, it would seem that it is that liability must be based upon conduct which is socially unreasonable. The common thread woven into all torts is the idea of unreasonable interference with the interests of others.[1]*

---

*Reprinted from Prosser and Keaton on the Law of Torts, W. Keeton, ed., 5th ed, copyright 1984, with permission of the West Publishing Corporation. This quotation and others that follow are acknowledged in the individual reference citations.

Interference with the interests of others may include activities or circumstances that may cause various harms, including death, bodily harm, disfigurement, disability, loss of income, loss of earning capacity, other items of financial loss or expense, damage to property, damage to reputation, alienation of affections, infliction of mental suffering, infliction of pain, or disruption of familial relationships. Though physicists may be sued for a civil wrong, a tort, generally they can not be accused of a crime resulting from purely professional actions. However, one can conceive of a physicist being accused of theft, fraud, criminal negligence, or perjury. We will not deal with these criminal possibilities but will focus on tort law.

> The early law of torts was not concerned primarily with the moral responsibility or "fault" of the wrongdoer. It occupied itself chiefly with keeping the peace between individuals, by providing a remedy which would be accepted in lieu of private vengeance.[2]

The law of tort had its birth in early English common law. It is a reasonable body of jurisprudence created by a civilized society to provide a peaceful, fair, and impartial allocation of losses arising from human activity. Tort law is not static and at any given time roughly reflects the public policy and moral makeup of a country. As our society entered the Industrial Age of the nineteenth century, law in the United States favored industry and professionals over the average person. The pendulum began to swing against industry and professionals in favor of individuals in the early part of the twentieth century. The directional swing of the pendulum gained momentum after World War II but may be slowing today.

If there is sufficient need, the law may change in response to lay people's belief that it is unjust in one area or another. However, the law does not change easily. Established legal principles set a precedent for the resolution of controversies in court and in countless controversies out of court, which makes predictability important. In the court systems, novel interpretations of substantive law, rules of procedure, and rules of evidence are often first formulated by judges in trial courts and then approved or rejected by the appropriate intermediate appellate or supreme courts. Thus, the civil justice system is a dynamic, living system that conserves elements that have worked in the past but also allows for changes on an ongoing basis. Common law (or judge-made law) is usually narrowly related to the controversy at hand. Statutes passed by legislatures are often broadly drawn and may alter the legal landscape in accordance with the wishes of the legislators and ultimately the voting citizens.

When changes in the law occur there are often winners and losers, who usually have opposite opinions on the merit of the changes. Currently, many business people and professionals think of tort law as an instrument for the redistribution of wealth rather than an instrument of just compensation for injured persons.[3] In the late 1980s, West Virginia State Judge R. Neely said:

> Liability law is a massive, off-line, wealth-redistribution program that enjoys overwhelming popular support yet many of us who administer the liability law are coming to understand that . . . something should be done about it before its unhappy consequences become all too apparent . . . .[4]

In some counties in Texas, large awards in personal injury cases are routinely granted. The defendants are usually large corporations or insurance companies headquartered at a distance but doing business in a county. Some corporations have withdrawn from one county completely; others are reluctant to hire local residents. In the late 1980s a railroad pulled up all its tracks in the county. The unemployment rate in that county is now more than twice the Texas average. However, these selected comments do not prove that lawsuits reduce economic activity.

Moderation in damage awards could come if juries begin to realize that the average citizen eventually pays for large damage awards in the cost of services, insurance premiums, or even lost jobs. Institutions upon which those citizens depend, such as hospitals, may be forced to diminish service or even seek bankruptcy protection. Sensitivity to the detrimental effect of a trial on a hospital was shown by plaintiffs in MacKay v. St. Charles Medical Center (1991). A miscalibration of a linear accelerator resulted in 592 patients receiving 13% to 14% more radiation than prescribed. The plaintiffs wanted to have separate trials for the health care professionals and the hospital because otherwise "a local jury would then be asked to bring in a verdict that would affect their local hospital."[5] The hospital asked for the right to participate as one of the defendants in the same, single trial unless plaintiffs agreed not to assert vicarious liability (employer liable for actions of employee) against the hospital on the basis of negligence of the other defendants. The plaintiffs did not agree. However, the trial court allowed the hospital to be part of a single trial, and the appeals court affirmed. The plaintiffs' lawyers believed that in this instance the jurors would balance the benefit of a damages award to the plaintiffs against the harm to the hospital and the community.

A medical malpractice lawsuit may cost the defendant or the insurers $50,000 or more just in defense costs and require three to five years of attention. The high cost and long delay of civil court actions brought into use a methodology called Alternative Dispute Resolution (ADR) for resolving disputes by mediation or arbitration. The methods of mediation and arbitration differ, but both seek to reduce the costs and accelerate the speed of resolving civil disputes. Judging by the amount of literature published and the number of legal short courses and seminars offered, this movement appears to be gaining acceptance. Busy trial judges and many litigants have enthusiastically used ADR. Yet some observers fear that it poses a threat to the traditional right to trial by jury. Perhaps we are at the beginning of a dynamic competition between methods of alternative dispute resolution and the civil court system. For more about ADR, see § 9.

The fear and perhaps hatred of the law that many may feel today obscures for them the importance and elegance of the legal structure, which through the turmoil of the adversary system brings forth the elements necessary for adjudicating a controversy. Our system makes it possible for real world adversaries to resolve real world disputes. We see a similarity between the functioning of the common law and physics or medical physics. Both are based upon experience to formulate principles that are then tested by new experience. New interpretations of the law are tested in the courts, and new theories in physics are tested by peers in refereed journals. Both build a structure of knowledge that attempts to be logically consistent. Both hold to established principles as long as possible in the face of new understanding or need, but both have mechanisms to accommodate change. The truth-defining mechanism in physics is the open corroboration of theory or experiment by peers. In the realm of common law, the truth-defining mechanism consists of decisions by trial courts, appellate courts, state supreme courts, and ultimately the U.S. Supreme Court.

§ 3   Changes in the Law—Tort Reform

A report of the Physicians Insurers Association of America, which consists of 33 physician-owned insurance companies, indicates that in 1995 24% of all patient claims and lawsuits were against diagnostic radiologists.[6] These claims correlated strongly with the increased use of mammography for breast cancer screening. The average payment to claimants stemming from the failure to diagnose breast cancer increased from $221,524 in 1990 to $301,460 in 1995. The cost to insurance companies for lawyers, expert witnesses, and administration was $28,700 per case in 1995. The report did not separate court cases from out-of-court settlements.

For the year ending June 30, 1992, there were 18,452 medical malpractice cases of all kinds in the nation's 75 most populous counties. Of these, 69.4% were resolved in an agreed settlement; 23.7% had summary judgments, default judgments, dismissal, or directed verdicts; and 6.9% had trial verdicts. Of the trial verdicts, 26% were in favor of the plaintiffs.[7]

In the mid 1970s, the number and dollar amounts of medical malpractice claims increased sharply. Many commercial insurance carriers withdrew either completely or selectively from the medical malpractice market, leaving a "crisis in availability" for liability insurance protection. Two responses to this crisis occurred. By 1983 at least 24 physician-owned insurance companies had been formed, and during the late 1970s 49 states had passed some sort of medical malpractice statute to make it more difficult to bring groundless lawsuits and to limit the costs of successful suits to defendants. However, by 1984, it was clear that these reforms had not had the effect intended.[8] The greatest weakness of the reform measures was that they were specific to medical liability cases and in large part were held unconstitutional piece by piece by state supreme courts. Plaintiffs were able to argue that their constitutional right to equal protection of the laws was violated. That is, patient-plaintiffs argued that the medical malpractice laws made it harder for them to file and win a lawsuit and recover damages than for plaintiffs in other types of lawsuits.

The courts then had to decide whether the unequal treatment of medical liability plaintiffs compared with other kinds of tort plaintiffs was justified. Thus, caps on damages, mandatory pretrial screening panels, and other parts of medical malpractice reform were susceptible to constitutional challenges in many states. Shortening the time limit for filing a lawsuit (§ 10) ran afoul of common law interpretations. Some of the reforms, such as fixing the percentage of the contingency fee for the plaintiff's lawyers, may have had the perverse effect of increasing the amount of damages sought. Under political attack by plaintiff lawyer groups, provisions in 12 states have been repealed or allowed to expire. However, some of the reforms have been notably successful in reducing costs in some states. Two examples are the changing of the collateral source rule, thus preventing a plaintiff from collecting for medical expenses redundantly from both health insurance and the defendant, and allowing the periodic payment of damages to successful plaintiffs who may die before collecting the full amount awarded.

During 1995, state legislatures debated more than 70 new tort bills. Bills applying to all torts may avoid the unconstitutionality trap of the 1970s medical malpractice bills. Between 1986 and 1995 various changes in basic tort law made by individual states included: replacement or alteration of joint and several liability so that a defendant having partial liability could not be forced to pay the full damages (41 states); some restriction of products liability (31 states); capping punitive damages (12 states); prohibiting punitive damages (4 states); requiring clear and convincing evidence, i.e., a higher standard, for punitive damages (17 states); capping non-economic damages (17 states); and changing the collateral source rule by reducing damages by amounts received in other compensation (8 states).[9]

Advocates for or against federal tort reform are very active in 1996. A federal statute would impose uniformity across the nation in this matter.

Whether to enact such a statute is a political question. On this question uncontradicted facts are few, and predictions of dire consequences, either way, are many. One prediction, however, seems quite sure—medical malpractice lawsuits will continue, and the impact of such suits upon defendant medical physicists will continue to be serious, regardless of whether or not new federal statutory laws come into being.

2

TYPES OF LAWSUITS

§ 4   Negligence

Negligence is a species of tort law based upon "fault." Fault is a departure from a standard of conduct required of a person by society for the protection of others. Fault in a tort context is not necessarily morally blameworthy; the conduct may not have been intended to cause harm but nonetheless failed to meet an accepted standard of conduct. That standard is often referred to as the "reasonable man" standard. For example, a man who has no intention or desire to cause any harm, but who is in some respect ignorant, misinformed, or careless, may do something or fail to do something and thereby cause harm to another person. This person may be liable to the injured party if a reasonable man, under the same or similar circumstances, would have done things differently and thereby avoided causing harm to that other person. The accepted standard of conduct changes with time. Professional conduct on the part of a medical physicist that may have been excusable ignorance 15 years ago may be regarded as negligent ignorance today. Negligence is a general legal theory applied across the spectrum of human activity. The following four elements are necessary to establish a claim of negligence (taken from Prosser and Keeton).[10]

1. A duty, or obligation, recognized by the law, requiring the actor to conform to a certain standard of conduct, for the protection of others from unreasonable risks. [Duty Defined by Standard of Care]

2. A failure on the part of the actor to conform to the standard required; a breach of the duty. [Breach of Duty]
3. A reasonably close causal connection between the conduct and the resulting injury. This is what is commonly known as "legal cause," or "proximate cause," and which includes the notion of cause in fact. [Cause of Injury]
4. Actual loss or damage resulting to the interest of another. [Damage]

In a jury trial, the judge, usually described as "the court," decides issues of law, and the jury decides issues of fact. The jurors will decide whether all the elements of negligence have been proven by a preponderance of the evidence (greater than 50%) to be more likely than not. If a plaintiff fails to prove one element of negligence, the plaintiff's case fails. To prove an issue by a preponderance of the evidence is a lesser burden of persuasion than that needed to prove an issue beyond reasonable doubt as required in criminal trials. Each of the elements of negligence is elaborated upon below.

Duty Defined by Standard of Care (Element 1): The duty of a physician to a patient is acquired in the establishment of the *doctor-patient relationship;* a hospital also has a duty of care to the patient that is sometimes called *direct corporate liability.* The duty of a medical physicist to a patient is usually derived from the duty of the physician or the hospital to the patient and is embodied in the terms or understanding of the physicist's employment. The existence of a duty on the part of a physician or a medical physicist is a question of law to be determined by the judge. The standard of conduct, usually called the standard of care in medical negligence cases, defines the duty of a medical professional to a patient in the case at hand and is a pivotal issue. Expert witnesses may receive intense questioning on this issue. The law generally holds the physician (or medical physicist) to the standard of care expected of a reasonable and prudent physician (or medical physicist) exercising ordinary care under the same or similar circumstances. This standard is consistent with traditional tort principles that hold a person of exceptional skill or knowledge to a duty of acting as would a reasonable and prudent person who possesses the same or similar skill or knowledge.[11, 12] Medical physicists and specialist physicians such as radiologists and radiation oncologists are held to a national standard of care.

A poor medical result, standing alone, is not proof of negligence. A practicing medical professional represents, either explicitly or by implication, that he or she has the training, knowledge, and skill of an ordinary, prudent practitioner of the same type and will apply these capabilities with reasonable care, diligence, and judgment. A physician may be held responsible for a mistake in judgment if he or she caused harm through failure to exercise the ordinary degree of care in making the judgment, which includes skill and diligence, of a physician of the same kind under similar circumstances. However, when a physician has exercised reasonable care and diligence in making a judgment, the physician will not be held liable for an error in that judgment. This is a well-established and long-standing principle, appearing, for example, in Texas cases in 1858 and 1964.[13]

Medical Physicists do not ordinarily exercise direct medical judgment in the care of patients, but there are some judgments that physicists are expected to make. If those judgments affect the care of a patient, the same type of general rule should apply to the physicist as to the physician. A mistake in measurement or calculation is not an error in judgment except under very unusual circumstances. Usually mistakes in radiation measurement or calculation that result in injury and damage to a patient will be found to be negligence on the argument that a safety net should have been in place to discover errors.

The general standard of care is a matter of law. Members of the jury do not get to choose the standard they would like to use. The defendant and expert witnesses present views of what actions were required by the particular standard of care appropriate to the case being adjudicated at the time of the alleged negligence (not at the time of trial). If reasonable persons could not differ in the determination of the standard of care, the judge (called the court) will make that determination as a matter of law; if reasonable persons could differ, the jury will weigh the facts presented within guidelines of law supplied by the judge. Judges will not question a jury's evaluation and finding of facts unless the evaluation and application are unreasonable. Judges rarely do this. Prosser has stated:

> While the function of the court, then, is primarily to determine the law, it must also decide some questions of fact, as to whether the evidence makes an issue sufficient for the jury; and the function of the jury in fixing the standard of reasonable conduct is so closely related to law that it amounts to a mere filling in of the details of the legal standard.[14]

The basis for determining the standard of care has evolved from a "customary" standard based on practices of similar medical professionals toward a more objective "good" standard. Though writers of texts and law reviews have usually shied away from using the term "minimum standard of care," a "good" standard logically must be a minimally acceptable standard.[15] Perdue has suggested that a modern standard of care for medical professionals should be based on what texts say, what professional schools teach, what other professionals do in their practices, what various professional organizations or boards recommend, what the expert witnesses recommend, and what the expert witnesses do in their own practice.[16] This combination of approaches includes what is "customary" as part, but only part, of the consideration. An important Washington state case, Helling v. Carey[17] demonstrates that a customary standard of care may be held inadequate. In that case the record showed without dispute that an ophthalmologist following the usual practice did not routinely test patients less than 40 years old for glaucoma. In a younger patient, the delay in discovery of the disease resulted in significant sight loss. The trial court found in favor of the defendant ophthalmologist on the basis of customary practice; the decision was affirmed by the appellate court. The state supreme court reversed, holding that the defendants were negligent as a matter of law for not routinely administering the simple and inexpensive glaucoma test to all patients. The court said:

> The precaution of giving this test to detect the incidence of glaucoma to patients under 40 years of age is so imperative that irrespective of its disregard by the standards of the ophthalmology profession, it is the duty of the courts to say who is required to protect patients under 40 from the damaging results of glaucoma.[18]

The duty of a medical physicist is not as clearly defined as that of a physician who has entered a physician-patient relationship. The responsibilities and the authority of a medical physicist may differ from institution to institution. For example, a medical physicist may be responsible for the correct fulfillment of radiation dose prescriptions at institution A but not at institution B. For further discussions of the medical physicist's duty and responsibilities see chapter four. Clearly, the standard of care applied to a medical physicist would have to allow for any boundaries placed upon the functioning of the physicist by the physicist's employer. It is better that these responsibilities be defined in writing before a patient incident. In court, the specific duty required by the standard of care for the medical physicist will be established by testimony that is usually supplied by both the plaintiff's and the defendant's expert witnesses.

Governmental Statutes and Regulations: Interestingly, a specific radiologic examination is the first medical procedure for which the federal government has legislated a national standard of care that enumerates specific duties. This standard of care is formulated in the Mammography Quality Standards Act (MQSA) of 1992.[19] It is likely that both plaintiff's attorneys and defendant's attorneys will use parts of MQSA requirements to argue their client's interests not only for mammography but also for other radiologic procedures.

What is the status of a statute or regulation in determining the standard of care in a particular lawsuit involving negligence? Fortunately, there is a long history of this issue in other activities that is applicable in medicine. A concise statement is given by Prosser:

> Where there is a normal situation, clearly identical with that contemplated by the statute or regulation, and no special circumstances or danger are involved, it may be found, and can be ruled as a matter of law, that the actor had done his full duty by complying with the statute, and nothing more is required. Thus, a railroad may not be required to protect a country crossing, with an unobstructed view, which is little used, by anything more than the statutory warning sign. But if there are unusual circumstances, or increased danger beyond the minimum which the statute was designed to meet, it may be found that there is negligence—and perhaps even recklessness— in not doing more.[20]

In Silkwood v. Kerr-McGee Corp. (1979) the employee of a nuclear fuel processing plant was found to have plutonium in her apartment.[21] The court held that compliance with government safety regulation could be accepted as evidence that Kerr-McGee Corp. had acted reasonably but should not be used as conclusive proof. This case illustrates that courts may find (wrongly in some cases) the existence of circumstances beyond those contemplated in the regulations and that the entire duty of the defendant is not met by complying with regulations. In O'Conner v. Commonwealth Edison Co. (1990) [22] a worker at a nuclear power plant was exposed to radiation when a flush of radioactive fluids passed through pipes nearby. Personal radiation monitors worn by the worker-plaintiff showed radiation exposure within limits set by the statute. The court accepted that the maximum permissible radiation dose levels set by federal safety standards provided the applicable standard of care. Thus, in this case the court found a normal situation contemplated by the statute or regulation with no special circumstances or danger. In a different case, Hernandez v. Nueces County Medical Soc. (1989),[23] a blood bank was accused of negligently failing to use two tests that could have detected a disease acquired by the plaintiff through a blood transfusion. These tests were not required by either the Federal Drug Administration or the American Association of Blood Banks. In this case, the court held that compliance with national regulatory standards did not establish the standard of care as a matter of law.[24] The omitted tests were used routinely by some blood banks and had been used occasionally by the defendants. Here the court believed that there was increased danger beyond the minimum standard set by the regulations.

If a medical physicist complies with a regulation, that regulation may fully define the standard of care expected for the activity addressed, but a higher standard could be defined and justified in a trial for negligence. If a physicist fails to comply with a regulation and that failure results in injury and damage to a person it is likely that the standard of care required would be that defined by the regulation. Regulations are valuable in defining dose limits in radiation protection. Performance based imaging quality regulations may help raise the general quality of imaging systems. In 1987 the Nuclear Regulatory Commission considered a document called "Comprehensive Quality Assurance in Medicine and a Standard of Care," relating to radiation therapy. This proposed rule was withdrawn because it was judged to be too onerous and restrictive. In its place regulations requiring reporting of radiation misadministrations were adopted in 1991 as discussed in § 40 below. Thus, regulations play a major role in defining the standard of care in radiation protection and a small but probably increasing role in defining the standard of care in imaging quality. In radiation therapy, regulations play essentially no role in defining the standard of care and are unlikely to do so because of the individualized nature of each treatment, the evolving methods of treatment, and the many treatment sites.

Breach of Duty (Element 2): After testimony regarding the standard of care in the instant case, arguments will be made on whether or not the defendant met an appropriate standard of care. To prevail, the plaintiff must establish that the defendant breached the standard of care. This is a fact issue determined by the jury.

Injury and Causation (Element 3): Causation in tort cases is an unsettled legal area that may never be fully delineated by rules. For negligence, the basis of causation is generally embodied in a concept called *proximate cause*. Included in proximate cause are "causation in fact" and "foreseeability." Basically, "causation in fact" means that injury to the plaintiff would not have occurred "but for" the actions or failure to act of the defendant. If there are multiple causes, the actions or failure to act of the defendant must have been a "substantial factor" in producing the injury to the plaintiff. Thus, the testimony of an expert witness might be sufficient to support a finding of causation if the expert stated that in his or her opinion *with reasonable medical probability* that the alleged conduct more likely than not was a cause of the harm.[25] Prosser and Keeton state:

> Once it is established that the defendant's conduct has in fact been one of the causes of the plaintiff's injury, there remains the question whether the defendant should be legally responsible for the injury . . . . [26] "Proximate cause" cannot be reduced to absolute rules. No better statement ever has been made concerning the problem than that of Street: "It is always to be determined on the facts of each case upon mixed considerations of logic, common sense, justice, policy and precedent."[27]

The kind of policy questions included in "proximate cause" include whether the defendant could reasonably foresee the injury to the plaintiff, whether the conduct of the defendant was unreasonable in proportion to the danger, whether there was an intervening cause that should be regarded as superseding the cause by the defendant, whether there is another person who had the duty of protecting the plaintiff, and whether there should be apportionment of liability among those responsible for various causes. In medical malpractice cases involving treatment, policy questions, for example, include consideration of preexisting conditions, asking whether the patient could have suffered the same medical results even if the alleged negligence had not occurred.

Alleged radiation injuries cover a wide spectrum. The bizarre end includes a recent case in which a woman alleged that her psychic powers were diminished or destroyed from x rays to the brain during a computerized axial tomography exam. Other types of late radiation injury, such as radiogenic cancer and genetic injury, have not been significant legal liabilities for the radiologist. This is fortunate because these suits are expensive and difficult to defend, even when they are frivolous.

Regarding late radiation injuries, in a 1992 statement The National Council on Radiation Protection and Measurements (NCRP) said:

> . . . it is not possible, on the basis of medical evaluation to unequivocally prove or disprove a claim that a specific malignancy was caused by a specified radiation exposure. [28]

The NCRP statement develops a probability of causation approach based upon probability, rather than proof to assign causation to an individual malignancy. However, in Radiation Injuries—Ionizing Radiation, Gooden[29] notes that the judiciary has a traditional abhorrence of statistical evidence. He also gives an extended discussion of late radiation injury in a radiation protection context, much of which is applicable to a malpractice claim involving late radiation injury. Of additional interest is NCRP Report No. 116,[30] which summarizes current radiation protection recommendations, including those relating to the protection of the embryo-fetus; Sinclair[31] gives the biological basis of those recommendations. The BEIR V Report[32] includes much background information.

In therapeutic radiology there is a narrow range of dose that produces enough radiation to achieve substantial benefit while introducing only acceptable risks. Radiation therapy can result in complications in 5% to 10% of patients even when done properly. This percentage of complications is accepted in order to improve the probability of a curative radiation dose. Patients should be counseled to accept the minor complications and not regard them as injury.

Until recently, diagnostic radiology incurred little legal liability for a missed or incorrect diagnosis. The reason for this was that the proximate cause of a patient's disease was not the missed diagnosis. For example, in the case of a missed lung cancer, the failure to diagnose the lung cancer was certainly not the cause of the cancer itself. However, the failure of a radiologist to diagnose a cancer or injury accurately and promptly may cost the patient a chance at cure or extended meaningful life. Public policy has shaped a legal response to this apparent injustice. It is referred to by several names, one of which is *lost chance due to delayed diagnosis.*

Radiologists are now being held legally liable for this lost chance in many but not all states. In fact, it is the greatest legal liability to radiologists today. The Physician Insurers Association of America's 1995 study of breast cancer[33] showed that malignant neoplasms of the female breast is the condition for which patients most often file a medical malpractice claim. This principle has affected radiologists in a profound manner; it may become significant to the diagnostic medical physicist in the future. Currently, radiologists are the specialists most frequently sued.

Poor-quality images have not been cited as a cause of a patient's injury in lawsuits. Yet, today's interest in performance-based standards may change this. The medical societies are producing performance-based standards of practice, and the MQSA is a performance-based federal law. It is reasonable to expect plaintiff's attorneys to attempt to link poor-quality images to a patient's lost chance due to delayed diagnosis. This may introduce new questions for the diagnostic medical physicist. Is a poor-quality image the result of an inadequate processor control program? Is a poor-quality image the result of too few physics evaluations of equipment? Is a poor-quality image the result of an inadequately trained technologist? Is a poor-quality image the result of some teleradiology operation or compression? Is the physicist responsible overall for the imaging quality?

Damage (Element 4): Proof of damage is an essential part of the plaintiff's case. Damages cannot be recovered for torts where no actual loss has occurred.[34]

Compensatory or actual damages in negligence malpractice cases may be sought by the patient for items including lost earnings and lost earning capacity, past, present, and future medical expenses, physical pain, and mental anguish. Members of the plaintiff's family can seek damages for loss of support, counsel, consortium, maintenance, companionship, household services, and past, present, and future mental suffering. Usually the plaintiff must have experienced physical injuries before related damages such as those listed above will be recognized.

Several tort law theories arising from common law and statutes are important in connection with claims alleging medical negligence. One is the doctrine from American common law of *joint and several liability,* which holds that a defendant may be held liable for all of an injured party's damages although the defendant contributed only partly to the injury. This theory provides an incentive for personal injury attorneys to seek "deep pocket" defendants. Attorneys may sue the pathologist, radiologist, surgeon, referring physician, medical physicist, hospital, and any other individual or entity that is even remotely associated with an alleged injury. As litigation progresses, defendants may be dismissed from the case based on their ability to pay rather than their culpability. As noted above under tort reform (§ 3), between 1986 and 1995 at least 41 states had abolished or modified joint and several liability in tort cases.

Another theory based on statutes is called comparative negligence. Until fairly recent times, tort law barred recovery of damages for the plaintiff whose own negligence contributed to the injury. This system favored defendants and was subject to abuse within the legal system. Courts in the United States recognized the inequity of this practice quite early, but found it difficult to fashion a different legal standard that could be adjudicated fairly. Today, however, all 50 states apply some form of comparative negligence or proportionate responsibility. In this situation, a defendant can be held responsible for a portion of damages (or in some states under certain conditions 100% of damages) even though a plaintiff contributed in significant measure to his or her own injury. A 1995 Texas statutory amendment states that a claimant may not recover damages if his or her percentage of responsibility is greater than 50 percent,[35] and if the claimant is not barred from recovery of damages, the amount of damages is reduced by the claimant's percentage of responsibility.[36, 37] However, in medical malpractice cases the defense of contributory negligence plays a minor role. Only negligent acts committed by the patient after becoming the defendant's patient may be construed as a contributing cause of injuries stemming from the malpractice.[38]

§ 5   Gross Negligence and Intentional Torts Resulting in Exemplary Damages

Gross Negligence: Attorneys will often seek exemplary (or punitive) damages in medical malpractice suits by claiming that not only was there negligence on the part of the physician and/or medical physicist but that there was gross negligence. Like many legal terms, gross negligence is difficult to define and has no generally accepted meaning. Prosser and

Keeton state that gross negligence "signifies more than ordinary inadvertence or inattention, but less perhaps than conscious indifference to the consequences."[39] Some might define gross negligence somewhat differently; for example, as an act or omission involving an extreme degree of risk to others and the actor, despite subjective awareness of the risk, proceeds in conscious indifference to the rights, safety, or welfare of others.[40, 41] Gross negligence may require proof by *clear and convincing evidence,* which is a standard greater than *preponderance of the evidence* required in most civil actions.[42]

Exemplary Damages: The terms exemplary damages and punitive damages are used interchangeably. (Exemplary damages is the preferred term.) However, there can be a slight distinction between them. Exemplary damages focus upon proper compensation for the plaintiff, and punitive damages focus on punishment of the defendant and deterrence of the defendant and others in the future. Physicists and physicians should be very concerned when gross negligence is plead in any lawsuit because *malpractice insurance may not cover awards of exemplary damages.* If the claim of gross negligence is frivolous, the defendant's attorney should seek to have it dismissed. If that pleading is not dismissed, it is litigated at trial. Exemplary damages were capped in a 1995 Texas statute to not exceed the greater of (a) two times the amount of economic damages (i.e., pecuniary loss) plus an amount equal to any non-economic damages not to exceed $750,000, found by the jury, or (b) $200,000.[43] These amounts may still seem large to a medical physicist on salary, but it is a retreat from the multi-million dollar awards possible earlier.

Changing of exemplary damages in tort cases by statute is always a heavily contended political issue. Similar political struggles are probably occurring in other states.

Intentional Torts: A physician can be accused of a number of types of intentional torts such as abandonment, battery (if the patient's consent for a procedure was not obtained), disclosure of confidential information, false imprisonment, or fraud (a misrepresentation of a material fact on which the patient relies, to his or her detriment).[44] Medical physicists are less likely than physicians to be involved in an intentional tort. However, disclosure of confidential information or fraud might be possible for a medical physicist.[45] All intentional torts are subject to exemplary damages.

3

LEGAL PROCEDURE

§ 9   Alternative Dispute Resolution

Before a suit is filed by a patient there may be significant opportunities to settle the dispute by informal means. Most patients want a health care professional to be fully honest with them about their treatment and to regard them with appropriate concern. There are remarkable stories about what medical mistakes patients have endured without legal recourse when they were treated honestly and well. Not charging for remedial treatment may be an important factor in resolving a dispute.

Alternative Dispute Resolution is a method of resolving medical malpractice disputes by mediation or arbitration. The main goals of Alternative Dispute Resolution are to resolve disputes more quickly and at less cost than in the court system. Mediation involves negotiating an agreement that is acceptable to both the plaintiff and the defendant; if an agreement is not reached by the parties, the mediation fails. The dispute can then go to trial or to some other type of dispute resolution. Arbitration is different from mediation in that once the plaintiff and defendant agree to the arbitration process, a binding determination will be made by an arbiter. This determination will have the weight of a court decision.

More than two-thirds of the states allow health insurers to ask patients to sign mediation or arbitration agreements. Less serious injuries that might not reach the court system may be entering alternative dispute resolution, thus increasing the number of claims. However, the settlements appear to be smaller. Neither mediation nor arbitration proceedings are public.

§ 10   Time Limit for a Lawsuit

A statute of limitations sets the amount of time within which a party must take judicial action or else lose the right to sue. Statutes of limitation were created to avoid lost evidence, failing memories, and staleness caused by the passage of time. In many states the applicable statute of limitation for medical malpractice is the same as that for other torts. Usually a malpractice suit must be filed within two years of the breach of duty that caused the alleged injury. However, a two-year statute of limitation favored defendants and under some circumstances put plaintiffs at significant disadvantages. For example, an injury caused by medical malpractice might not be discovered for months or even years after the original negligence. Now, most states have doctrines in place for malpractice torts that cause the statute of limitations to start running once the negligent injury is, or should have been, discovered by the plaintiff. There are also some other exceptions to starting the limitations period from the date of the injury that may be plead successfully by the plaintiff in some jurisdictions. Pleas for such suspension can be made (1) for plaintiffs who are minors until they reach a specified age, (2) until completion of the health care treatment or hospitalization, (3) because of fraudulent concealment of the patient's condition by the physician, (4) for the period of plaintiff imprisonment, (5) because of plaintiff insanity, (6) because of the absence of the defendant from the jurisdiction, or (7) for a specified period after the death of the plaintiff.

In actual practice, the statute of limitations may be determined by a combination of the state statutory law and judicial rulings. Probably most malpractice cases fall within the appropriate statute of limitations, but for exceptions that delay the statute, the services of a lawyer may be required. Thus, if a medical physicist is sued for negligence after the limitations period has expired, the physicist's lawyer should seek a summary judgment prior to a trial (§ 13). Also, if one of the defendants disappears, the period in which a plaintiff may bring a suit is extended. This event happened in a case discussed (§ 26).

§ 11   Expert Witnesses in Medical Malpractice Lawsuits

Medical physicists may appear in court as expert witnesses, particularly in medical malpractice cases where radiation dose is an issue. The expert witness is asked to participate by either the plaintiff's or the defendant's lawyer. Often the expert will communicate only with the lawyer, and not with the plaintiffs, defendants, or other experts. Early communications may be verbal to avoid discovery (forced production of documents for the information of the other side). Late in the pretrial process there may be a deposition of the expert recorded under oath at which calculations, graphs, or other documents prepared by the expert will be entered as evidence. Be aware that any material an expert brings to a deposition, including scribbled preliminary notes, may become an exhibit to the deposition if required by the opposing side. Also be aware that the opposing lawyers have full opportunity for questioning at a deposition. Before an expert can testify in court, the judge will hear of his or her education and experience and qualify the person as an expert witness. At trial the expert may be called to testify, or the deposition may be read into the record preserving the testimony from the deposition. In some states, depositions may be taken with the aid of a video recorder so that prior testimony can be seen and heard by the jury without the expert appearing in court.

What is the status and role of an expert witness? Testimony by a qualified expert is permitted when some body of knowledge or experience is technically beyond the common understanding of the layperson, and the expert, properly prepared for the case, offers opinions that are helpful to the jury. Lay witnesses may testify on what they have heard, seen, or otherwise observed, but the expert witness may go further to draw conclusions from evidence. In many trials, an expert witness will be asked to draw conclusions from a hypothetical question that includes, as assumptions, facts in evidence for the case being tried. However, the testimony of medical physicists often pertains to radiation dose and usually does not include hypothetical questions. In a negligence case, expert witnesses for the plaintiff or defendant will be called on to help establish what the national standard of care was at the time of the patient's diagnosis or treatment. The expert will be asked whether that standard was adhered to in the present case.

In a malpractice case in which a physician is the defendant, an expert witness who testifies on the standard of care will usually be a physician of the same specialty. However, physicists or other nonphysicians may be allowed to testify on the medical standard of care if they have adequate experience in the area to qualify as experts.[55] A physicist's testimony is likely to be admissible particularly if the radiation dose delivered is much more or much less than that prescribed or recommended in radiotherapy texts. However, the medical physicist who testifies on the medical standard of care can expect strenuous cross-examination about his or her experience and lack of medical credentials. A physician-expert may be asked if the breach of the standard of care to a *reasonable medical probability* caused the patient's injuries. In general, experts are expected to give their opinions in scientific or medical phraseology rather than in legal terms. For the defense, a physicist who is called as an expert witness might testify regarding standard of care, dose, and the appropriateness of the defendant's behavior (adherence to the standard of care and professional standards).

The process of testifying can be an interesting and professionally satisfying experience for a person called to be an expert witness. In a limited time the thoroughness of preparation, the skill of explanation, and the credibility of the individual as an expert is tested in an atmosphere of high drama and tension. The experience has a unique intensity.

§ 12   Evidence and How It May Be Presented

What constitutes acceptable evidence and when and how it may be presented before and during a trial is an issue that has a long history. Innovations occur from time to time to meet new circumstances in trials; the state supreme court decides to affirm new rules or allow changes to old rules of evidence for the state courts. These rules of evidence are in place to ensure the efficient presentation of sound and fair evidence. Objection to the introduction of evidence at trial may be made by the opposing attorney; the judge decides what can and cannot be presented into evidence in accordance with the rules of evidence. *Relevant evidence* is evidence having a tendency to make the existence of a fact of consequence more or less probable than it would be without the evidence. *Materiality* means that the evidence must be offered to prove a matter at issue. Evidence, oral or written, is *hearsay* when its probative or proving force depends in whole or in part on the competency and creditability of a person other than the witness.[56] A witness is not permitted to offer hearsay as evidence unless the evidence is offered under a hearsay exception.

If a medical physicist is a party in a lawsuit, the attorney will advise him or her on issues regarding evidence. Here we will focus on those aspects of evidence that may influence a medical physicist in the practice of medical physics or may be important in a lawsuit. The following rules of evidence or extracts are from the Federal Rules of Evidence (1995)[57] and the Texas Rules of Civil Evidence (1995)[58] when the Texas rule of evidence does not have a federal counterpart. Other states will have similar rules, but before relying upon the statements below the reader is advised to check the rules in the applicable jurisdiction.

Cannot Refuse to Testify: "No person has a privilege to (1) refuse to be a witness, or (2) refuse to disclose any matter, or (3) refuse to produce any object or writing, or (4) prevent another from being a witness or disclosing any matter or producing any object or writing" (partial Texas Rule 501).

Burden of Proof: The Burden of Proof has two distinct parts. *The Burden of Persuasion,* or establishing a proposition against all counterargument or evidence, resides with the plaintiff-patient in a medical malpractice case. *The Burden of Going Forward with the Evidence,* or presenting evidence to support a claim, resides initially with the plaintiff. However, this responsibility may shift to the defendant if a reasonable member of the jury could find the facts of the plaintiff's pleadings true. Thus, a defendant physicist may be in the position of trying to prove that the prescribed radiation dose was delivered to a target volume and that other structures were not over-irradiated. Dosimetry systems and programs should be designed so that they can be used in the physicist's defense. For example, independent verification of crucial steps, such as radiation machine calibration, is persuasive (see chapter five and § 23).

Best Evidence: "To prove the content of a writing, recording, or photograph, the original writing, recording, or photograph is required except as otherwise provided in these rules or by Act of Congress" (Federal Rule 1002). The original is not required, and other evidence of the contents of a writing, recording, or photograph is admissible if the original is lost or destroyed, not obtainable, in the possession of opponent, or is not closely related to a controlling issue (from Federal Rule 1004).

Records of Regularly Conducted Activity: "The following are not excluded by the *hearsay* rule, even though the declarant is available as a witness: a memorandum, report, record, or data compilation, in any form, of acts, events, conditions, opinions, or diagnoses, made at or near the time by, or from information transmitted by, a person with knowledge, if kept in the course of a regularly conducted business activity, and if it was the regular practice of that business activity to make the memorandum, report, or data compilation, all as shown by the testimony of the custodian or other qualified witness, unless the source of information or the method or circumstances of preparation indicate lack of trustworthiness. The term "business" as used in this paragraph includes business, institution, association, profession, occupation, and calling of every kind whether or not conducted for profit" (Federal Rule 803 [6]). Medical and physics records, such as radiation machine calibrations or tests of imaging quality, are included in this hearsay exception. To indicate trustworthiness, the records should be orderly and in ink or printed. If records are handwritten, recording in a bound book enhances the reliability of the record dates.

Recorded Recollection: "The following are not excluded by the hearsay rule, even though the declarant is available as a witness: a memorandum or record concerning a matter about which a witness once had personal knowledge but now has insufficient recollection to enable him to testify fully and accurately, shown to have been made or adopted by the witness when the matter was fresh in the witness' memory and to reflect that knowledge correctly. If admitted, the memorandum or record may be read into evidence but may not itself be received as an exhibit unless offered by an adverse party" (Federal Rule 803 [5]). Notes reflecting conversations with patients and physicians or written memoranda explaining changes in radiation machine calibration, correction of machine performance, correction of discovered errors of calculation, or anything affecting the fulfillment of radiation dose prescription may be important in a later legal action. Such written records also build confidence in the dosimetry system on the part of medical professionals who rely upon it.

Out-of-Court Experiments: Evidence from experiments conducted outside the courtroom is often admissible if the experiments are demonstrated to be relevant to the case. For example, measurements could be made on a phantom, simulating the treatment of a particular patient. The defendant has an advantage in such experiments because treatment conditions can be duplicated closely. Use of a properly qualified outside expert who is not a party in the case lends credibility to these efforts. Generally, courts will admit experimental evidence and not require notice to the opponent that such experiments are being conducted.

Scientific Evidence: The judge may accept relevant scientific evidence as given by an expert, depending upon the qualification of the expert and the general acceptance of the type of evidence by the scientific community.

Learned Treatises: "The following are not excluded by the hearsay rule, even though the declarant is available as a witness: to the extent called to the attention of an expert witness upon cross-examination or relied on by him in direct examination, statements contained in published treatises, periodicals, or pamphlets on a subject of history, medicine, or other science or art, established as a reliable authority by the testimony or admission of the witness or by other expert testimony or by judicial notice. If admitted, the statements may be read into evidence but may not be received as exhibits" (Federal Rule 803 [18]). Thus, published materials may be referred to in testimony if the source is credible. A search of pertinent literature is advisable for parties to a suit and for expert witnesses.

Impeaching a Witness: Impeaching the witness should more correctly be called impeaching the testimony of the witness. Nothing happens to the witness, but the testimony of the witness may have doubt cast upon its validity or creditability. Impeachment of witnesses generally occurs on cross-examination and involves an exposure of bias or prejudice or deficiencies in the expert's basic qualifications or preparatory work in a specific case. A witness being impeached may be confronted with prior inconsistent statements, particularly from his or her publications, testimony, or depositions in the current or other cases. A witness's previous statements are generally inadmissible except when offered to rebut a charge of recent fabrication. An expert witness may be asked how much he or she is being paid, whether the remuneration is dependent upon the outcome of the case, how frequently the expert testifies, and for which side.

Payment of Medical Expenses or Similar Expenses: "Evidence of furnishing or offering or promising to pay medical, hospital, or similar expenses occasioned by an injury is not admissible to prove liability for the injury" (Federal Rule 409). This policy is long established in common law and is not limited to medical malpractice cases; it encourages resolution of a disagreement without prejudicing possible later legal action.

Compromise and Offers to Compromise: "Evidence of (1) furnishing or offering or promising to furnish, or (2) accepting or offering or promising to accept, a valuable consideration in compromising or attempting to compromise a claim which was disputed as to either validity or amount is not admissible to prove liability for, or invalidity of the claim or its amount. Evidence of conduct or statements made in compromise negotiation is likewise not admissible" (partial Federal Rule 408). In short, efforts to resolve a dispute cannot be used to prove liability.

Liability Insurance: "Evidence that a person was or was not insured against liability is not admissible upon the issue whether he acted negligently or otherwise wrongfully. This rule does not require the exclusion of evidence of insurance against liability when offered for another purpose, such as proof of agency, ownership, or control, or bias or prejudice of a witness" (Federal Rule 411). Thus, the jury usually does not know whether or not the defendant has liability insurance. However, there may be instances in which the existence of insurance may be used as evidence of an employer-employee or principal-agent relationship.

Subsequent Remedial Measures: "When, after an event, measures are taken which, if taken previously, would have made the event less likely to occur, evidence of the subsequent remedial measures is not admissible to prove negligence or culpable conduct in connection with the event" (partial Federal Rule 407). Thus, if after a suit was initiated a medical physicist purchased a new imaging phantom for diagnostic radiology or subscribed to a service for testing radiation machine calibration by mailed dosimeters, this information could not be used to prove that the prior methods were negligent.

Notification of Defect: "A written notification by a manufacturer of any defect in a product produced by such manufacturer to purchasers thereof is admissible against the manufacturer on the issue of existence of the defect to the extent that is relevant" (Texas Rule 407 [b]).

Lawyer-Client Privilege: "A client has a privilege to refuse to disclose and to prevent any other person from disclosing confidential communication made for the purpose of facilitating the rendition of professional legal services to the client . . . ." (partial Texas Rule 503 [b]). Thus, if a medical physicist has been sued and has engaged a lawyer, information communicated to the lawyer is confidential.

Peer Privilege: Federal Rule 501 is a general rule of evidence concerning privileges. It states in part, ". . . the privilege of . . . a person . . . shall be governed by the principles of the common law as they may be interpreted by the courts of the United States in the light of reason and experience." In Texas, for example, all parties in a malpractice suit can obtain copies of the claimant's medical records or records made in the regular course of business, but the records and proceedings of a medical committee of a hospital or a committee appointed ad hoc to conduct a specific investigation are confidential and are not subject to court subpoena.[59] Further, incident reports of events inconsistent with routine procedure or treatment, even if the incident gives rise to a malpractice suit, are exempt from discovery if the report is a communication among agents, representatives, and employees of a party to litigation.[60] This privilege of internal communication is necessary to allow hospitals to understand unusual incidents and to correct procedures without endangering their position as a defendant in a malpractice case. The privilege is protected by case law and various state and federal statutory pronouncements. It may vary to some extent in different jurisdictions.

Trade Secrets: "A person has a privilege, which may be claimed by him or his agent or employee, to refuse to disclose and to prevent other persons from disclosing a trade secret owned by him, if the allowance of the privilege will not tend to conceal fraud or otherwise work injustice. When disclosure is directed, the judge shall take such protective measure as the interests of the holder of the privilege and of the parties and the furtherance of justice may require" (Texas Rule 507). For example, if a physicist has created a computer program that is relevant to a suit, proprietary information concerning the program may be protected.

Physician-Patient Privilege: "Confidential communications between a physician and a patient, relative to or in connection with any professional services rendered by a physician to the patient are privileged and may not be disclosed . . . Exceptions to the confidentiality or privilege in court or administrative proceedings exist (1) when the proceedings are brought by the patient against a physician, including but not limited to malpractice proceedings . . . (2) when the patient or someone authorized to act on his behalf submits a written consent to the release of any privileged information . . . . Any person who received information made privileged by this rule may disclose the information to others only to the extent consistent with the authorized purposes for which consent to release the information was obtained" (partial Texas Rule 509). Thus, a medical physicist who has confidential information about a patient should treat that information with the same regard as required of a physician.

§ 13   Procedure before Trial

The intent of civil legal procedure is to provide formal steps for the just and efficient settlement of legal controversies. Rules of civil procedure are formulated by the states and federal government with revisions as the need arises from trial experience. The Texas Rules of Civil Procedure with annotations (arising mostly from case law and reference to federal rules) comprise nine volumes. Similar rules exist in other states. The lawyer negotiates the procedural hurdles so a defendant medical physicist generally does not need to know this area of the law. However, we will briefly describe procedure before, during, and after trial.

A plaintiff initiates a legal action by filing an original petition called the plaintiff's pleading or complaint, which names the defendant or defendants, states the facts upon which the claim is based, and prays for relief (usually a monetary award). An appropriate state court is one that has subject matter and monetary jurisdiction, usually in the county where the act or omission occurred or where the defendant resides. A case may be tried in federal court when the plaintiff and the defendants are residents of different states. The federal court will apply the laws of the state in which it is located. In response to the plaintiff's pleading, the defendant files an answer, also called a pleading. A defendant's answer may object to the jurisdiction of the court, make a motion to change the venue or place of the trial, raise special exceptions to the form or substance of the plaintiff's pleadings, plead lack of capacity of parties to sue or be sued, plead affirmative defenses such as plaintiff assumed risk, and deny the plaintiff's pleadings. A defendant may also assert a cause of action against a third party who may be liable to the plaintiff for all or part of the plaintiff's claim against the defendant. Plaintiff's and defendant's pleadings may be amended in supplemental pleadings.

Pretrial discovery procedures are used to find facts and develop a case. Both the plaintiff and defendant may receive written questions, called *interrogatories,* which must be responded to under oath with an answer or objection. *A Request for Admissions* is a device for simplifying the trial by agreeing upon uncontradicted matters. *Production of Tangible Things* provides for the production of documents and other things for copying or photographing from parties or from non-parties with the court's permission. For example, in Texas, knowledge of insurance agreements, including policy limits and coverage, is allowed under the rules of discovery even though this information cannot be presented to the jury. The written reports of experts are discoverable; it is for this reason that early in a suit lawyers often want oral reports, which then become part of the work product of the attorney and are not discoverable by the other side.

Another part of the pretrial proceedings, depositions under oath may be responses to written or oral questions with full opportunity for cross-examination. At the time of deposition, the calculations or other written work by an expert are discoverable and may be entered as exhibits to the deposition. The depositions may be read into the trial record as evidence and may also be used to impeach the expert at trial if there is inconsistency between the expert's deposition and the trial testimony. Video recording of depositions sometimes supplements the recorded transcript and may be displayed to the jury in some states. A pretrial conference conducted by the judge who may try the case is effective in focusing issues and identifying evidence that will not be admitted.

A *default judgment* may be rendered against a defendant who has had proper service of citation and fails to answer in the required time. The trial court has rather broad discretion in setting aside a default judgment but has a limited amount of time to act before the judgment becomes final. A judge may order a new trial in a case in which the failure of the defendant to answer before judgment was neither intentional nor the result of conscious indifference on his or her part but due to a mistake or accident. However, the motion for a new trial must set a meritorious defense and be filed at a time so as not to inflict a hardship on the plaintiff. A medical physicist who is named as a defendant among other defendants in a legal action should ensure that the answer to the court is on time and includes his or her name. An interlocutory or temporary default judgment may be filed against a non-responding defendant even though the cause remains undisposed as to other defendants for whom timely answer has been filed.

A *summary judgment* based on pretrial written pleadings, interrogations, depositions, admissions, and affidavits may be requested by either party with the statement that there is no dispute of the facts. For example, when a defendant in a medical malpractice suit establishes that the time set by the statute of limitations has passed without circumstances that would delay the statute, the defendant is entitled to a summary judgment (see § 10). A summary judgment allows the judge to render the judgment without a jury trial.

§ 14   Trial Procedure

State constitutions guarantee the right to a jury trial in civil actions. In a jury trial, the judge decides matters of law, and the jury decides matters of fact. If the parties elect to have a non-jury trial, the judge will decide both matters of law and matters of fact. Jury selection is a very important part of a trial. An examination of each prospective juror determines whether he or she can be challenged, or not chosen, for cause such as bias or relationship to the parties. In addition, each side can challenge a specific number of prospective jurors without cause.

Ordinarily the plaintiff opens and closes the final argument. At the request of either party, witnesses who are not themselves parties may be placed under the "rule," which means they cannot hear other testimony.

A *directed verdict* may be called for if one party fails to present sufficient evidence to uphold the case. The judge will require the jury to decide in favor of the opposing party. The defendant may move for a directed verdict at the end of the presentation of the plaintiff's evidence, and either party may so move at the end of all the evidence. A directed verdict by the judge to the jury is proper only when there is no evidence upon which the nonmoving party can win; if reasonable minds could differ on this question, a directed verdict is not proper, and the case is submitted for jury consideration.

§ 15   Procedure after a Trial

After a verdict by the jury either party may move for a judgment. The party favored by the verdict will move for *judgment on the verdict.* The other party may move for a new trial for various reasons such as erroneous evidentiary rulings by the judge, irreconcilable findings on issues by the jury, jury misconduct, newly discovered evidence, jury finding against the weight of the evidence, and inadequate or excessive damages. The trial court, i.e., the judge, may render a judgment on the verdict or grant a new trial but may also render a judgment contrary to the jury verdict. If there is no reasonable evidence supporting the verdict or if the jury verdict is contrary to law, the trial judge may affirm a motion for *judgment notwithstanding the verdict.* If the damages in the verdict are greater than the plaintiff has requested, contrary to statute, or otherwise excessive, the trial judge (in response to a motion by the defendant) may offer the plaintiff a choice of lesser damages or a new trial *(remittitur).*

The party not favored by the verdict may appeal the decision to the appropriate court if the lawyer contested an error in the trial at the time it occurred. To be reversible, the error must have been such that it was calculated to cause and probably did cause, the rendition of an improper judgment. For example, if the plaintiff's attorney informed the jury that the defendant had liability insurance, this would undoubtedly be a basis for reversing a judgment in favor the plaintiff if it was objected to by the defendant's attorney at the time. The appellate court may fully affirm or fully reverse the judgment of the trial court, remand all or part of the case to the trial court for a new trial, or suggest reduction of the amount of damages. In the latter instance, the party awarded the judgment has a choice of accepting the reduced amount or enduring a new trial (remittitur).

A final judgment that is not appealed or that survives an appeal is a settled issue that cannot be relitigated in a new cause of action *(res judicata).* This finality is in accord with the two objectives of the adjudicative process that are often in conflict. The first is to see that substantial justice is done on the merits, and the second is to bring legal controversy to a final conclusion with reasonable promptness and cost.[61]

§16   A Medical Physicist Encounters the Law (2) (Story continued from §1)

The plaintiff's original petition to the court accompanied the summons given to Barbara Hickman. An abbreviated amended petition is given here. The defendants' answer to the court was required within a fixed time following the arrival of the summons. An abbreviated amended defendants' answer is also given. Note the legal style.

<u>PLAINTIFF'S FIFTH AMENDED PETITION</u>

After identifying the parties, the petition stated that the district court in the county had jurisdiction and venue, that the defendants had been served with process, had answered, and are before this court in all respects.

I.
<u>PHYSICIAN-PATIENT RELATIONSHIP AND HOSPITAL PATIENT RELATIONSHIP</u>
At all times material herein plaintiff STIFLER had a physician-patient relationship with defendant BREWSTER and a hospital-patient relationship with defendant MOUNTAIN VIEW RADIATION CENTER and defendant HICKMAN as an employee of defendant MOUNTAIN VIEW RADIATION CENTER or as a borrowed servant of defendant BREWSTER owed a duty of care to plaintiff STIFLER.

II.
<u>STATEMENT OF FACTS</u>
Plaintiff was referred to the radiation center for radiation treatment of squamous cell carcinoma of the left eyebrow and left upper eyelid. After numerous radiation treatments the plaintiff developed significant discomfort in the affected eye area. The plaintiff complained to the defendants of pain and discomfort and also a decrease in vision and irritation of the eye. It became apparent that the plaintiff had sustained severe and profound damage to the eye due to excessive radiation used in treatment. The defendants, and each of them, carelessly and negligently and through gross negligence committed acts and/or omissions amounting to a failure to possess and/or exercise and comply with that degree of knowledge, skill and care ordinarily and reasonably possessed by other physicians and medical physicists specializing in radiation oncology in the same or similar circumstances as follows:

a. In failing to protect the eye from the effects of radiation;
b. In failing to limit radiation treatments to a safe level;

c. *In failing to use eye shields around the eye in the proper manner to protect the plaintiff's eye; and*

d. *In using an improper type of radiation (electrons) which is never used anywhere for the treatment of plaintiff's condition, rather than low energy x ray.*

All of the above acts or omissions by defendants, either independently or in conjunction with each other, constituted negligence and gross negligence and were proximate cause of plaintiff's injuries and damages described herein.

WHEREFORE, PREMISES CONSIDERED, Plaintiff prays that defendants be cited to appear and answer herein and after a final hearing hereon that plaintiff have:

1. *Judgment against defendants as follows:*
    a. *Past pain and suffering in an amount of $500,000.00*
    b. *Future pain and suffering in an amount of $500,000.00*
    c. *Past mental anguish in an amount of $375,000.00*
    d. *Future mental anguish in an amount of $375,000.00*
    e. *Past physical impairment in an amount of $1,000,000.00*
    f. *Future physical impairment in an amount of $1,000,000.00*
    g. *Past disfigurement in an amount of $50,000.00*
    h. *Future disfigurement in an amount of $50,000.00*
    i. *Past medical expenses in an amount of $5,000.00*
    j. *Future medical expenses in an amount of $50,000.00*
    k. *Exemplary damages in an amount of $3,000,000.00*
2. *Pre-judgment interest on the amount accrued on the damage amount(s) at the highest legal rate allowed by law;*
3. *Post-judgment interest on the due amount at the highest legal rate from the date of judgment until paid; and*
4. *That plaintiff recover all costs of court.*

Attorneys for Plaintiff

DEFENDANTS' FIRST AMENDED ORIGINAL ANSWER

After identifying the court, the case, and the parties, parts of the answer pertinent here are given.

I.

Defendants deny each and every, all and singular, the allegations in the plaintiff's petition pleadings contained, and demand strict proof thereof.

II.

Answering further, and in the alternative, and by way of affirmative defense, if that be necessary, these defendants would show that use of electron beam treatment for malignancies of the eyelid and regions around the eye is a long established conventional treatment and where bone underlies the treated area, as in this case, is superior to low-energy x-ray treatment.

III.

Furthermore, and in the alternative, and by way of affirmative defense, if that be necessary, defendants would show that the proximate or producing or legal cause, either solely or in part, of the harms and damages complained of herein by plaintiff, if any, was the negligence or fault or contributory or comparative negligence or fault of plaintiff himself. The plaintiff upon his own initiative exposed himself to the improper use of corticosteroids including diprolene, diprosone and aristocort, by using these on and/or in and/or around the area of the left eye and left upper eyelid after the radiation treatments of the plaintiff by the defendants complained of in the plaintiff's petition when such use was improper and likely to cause severe damage.

IV.

Answering further, and in the alternative, and by way of affirmative defense, if that by necessary, defendants would show that imposition of punitive or exemplary damages would be fundamentally unfair and would violate the constitution of the United States and the Constitution of this state.

V.

Answering further, and in the alternative, and by way of affirmative defense, if that be necessary, and as a matter of law, defendants would show that the new statutory definition of "gross negligence" in this state's Civil Practice and Remedies Code requires of a plaintiff at least a "clear and convincing" standard of proof which is a standard greater than the "preponderance of evidence" standard.

WHEREFORE, PREMISES CONSIDERED, these defendants pray that the plaintiff take nothing by reason of this suit, that these defendants recover their costs expended, and for all such other and further relief, at law and equity, to which they may be justly entitled under the law, the evidence and their pleadings properly on file herein, and shall ever so pray.

Attorney for Defendants

(This story is continued in § 35.)

4

THE LEGAL DUTY OF MEDICAL PHYSICISTS

§ 17 Origin of Legal Duty of Medical Physicists

A physician in private practice is an independent contractor who acquires responsibility to a patient through formation of the physician-patient relationship. The physician-patient relationship usually involves an expressed or implied contractual agreement whereby the physician offers to treat the patient with proper professional skill, and the patient agrees to pay for such treatment.[62] However, once a physician-patient relationship is commenced, society imposes a duty of care upon the physician through tort law (§4). A majority of jurisdictions regard a physician as an independent contractor if the physician is chosen by the patient. Physicians who are independent contractors are responsible for their own actions, the actions of their employees, and the actions of hospital employees whom they control as *borrowed servants.* The older *captain of the ship* doctrine in which a physician, particularly a surgeon, was responsible for everything that occurred is invoked rarely today. In Baird v. Sickler[63] (1982) the court made "no attempt to impose upon an operating physician the duty of overseeing all that occurs in the highly technical milieu in which he works." Further discussion is given by King.[64] If a physician is the employee or otherwise the agent of the hospital or is the apparent agent (ostensible agent) of the hospital as perceived by the patient, the duty of the physician may derive in some way from the duty of the hospital to the patient.   ·

Until about 30 years ago hospitals were regarded essentially as hotels that provided housing for independent contractor physicians and their patients. Increasingly, hospitals became involved in the delivery of health care, providing specialized facilities, various skilled personnel, and overall supervision of the quality of health care delivered. Two overlapping legal theories that have evolved in case law are (1) *vicarious liability* for the negligence of hospital employees, agents, or apparent agents, and (2) *direct corporate liability* based on the concept that a hospital has a direct non-delegable duty of care to its patient. This duty includes liability for selecting proper and safe equipment, for exercising reasonable care in retaining and supervising independent contractors (physicians and probably physicists as well), and for negligently failing to adopt, to formulate adequately, or to supervise hospital rules and policies. For a fuller discussion see Perdue,[65] King[66] or Trail and Kelly-Claybrook.[67] Does a medical physicist have a legal duty to a patient? Prosser and Keeton state:

> No better general statement can be made than that the courts will find a duty where, in general, reasonable persons would recognize it and agree that it exists. [68]

This sentiment has been refined in case law defining the duty of physicians and hospitals toward patients. The beginning of duty for physicians and for hospitals is the agreement with the patient establishing a physician-patient or hospital-patient relationship.

Nurses, pathologists, and medical physicists do not have agreements with patients. The legal duty of nurses is more developed in case law than that of medical physicists and may indicate the direction of development of legal duty for medical physicists. Menges[69] states, ". . . a nurse's negligence, under agency principles, may be imputed to either the physician or surgeon in charge, the hospital employing the nurse, or to both or neither." Earlier cases, particularly, distinguished whether a nurse at the time of a negligent act was doing an administrative function for the hospital, such as transporting a patient, or a medical function for the physician, such as assisting in a surgical operation. However, there are times when a nurse does not have supervision from a physician or a hospital, such as in an industrial dispensary. In Baur v. Mesta Machine Co.[70] the court concluded that the standard required of registered nurses was that of "a reasonably prudent registered nurse in charge of an industrial dispensary" or, as in subsequent cases, wherever the nurse was working. In a 1983 Texas case, Lunsford v. Board of Nurse Examiners,[71] the court concluded that a nurse's duty to a patient stems from the nurse's state licensure and that the nurse had a legal duty to stabilize a patient's condition and prevent complications even though a physician instructed the nurse to send an emergency patient to another hospital. A pathologist has been held to have a physician-patient relationship with patients even though the pathologist performs diagnostic work and may not see the patient.[72]

The origin of the duty of a medical physicist who is negligent is of importance in determining who is liable for damages. If the duty of a medical physicist arises from the physician-patient relationship or the hospital-patient relationship, the physician or hospital would likely also be a defendant if the medical physicist is accused of negligence in a malpractice action. The employer is vicariously liable in an action based upon the physicist's negligence. However, be aware that an employer can seek *indemnification* from an employee, that is, repayment of amounts the employer paid in damages to a plaintiff for the negligent acts of the employee. Indemnification is available in cases where the liability of a defendant, e.g., an employer, arises through the action of law (here vicarious liability) rather than his or her own negligent actions. If the medical physicist's duty to a patient arises independently of a physician or a hospital, the liability for a negligent act may reside solely in the physicist. This situation may sometimes arise for medical physicists who are independent contractors. The duty of a medical physicist to a patient independent of the duty of a physician or a hospital to a patient is not explicitly developed in case law. However, most, and possibly all, medical physicists believe they have a duty to patients; patients who are aware of the activities of medical physicists probably also believe that medical physicists have a duty to them. With certainty, courts will find that medical physicists have a duty to patients whether that duty is derivative from a physician-patient relationship, a hospital-patient relationship, or if those relationships are not applicable, arises independently from a generalized tort theory developed for the case at hand.

If a physicist is not an employee, he or she may be the agent of a physician or hospital. An *agent* is one who acts for or in place of another by authority from the *principal*. The agent is a substitute, a deputy, appointed by the *principal* with power to do the things that the *principal* may do.[73] If that is the relationship, vicarious liability would still apply, and the principal, that is, the physician or hospital, would be liable for the physicist's negligence.

If a medical physicist is an independent contractor, the physicist may be liable for his or her own negligence and that of the physicist's employees. A contractor is one who makes an agreement with another to do a piece of work, retaining in himself or herself the control of means, method, and manner of producing the result to be accomplished. Neither party has the right to terminate the contract at will.[74] Whether a consulting medical physicist functionally is an agent or an independent contractor may not always be easily determined. A defining characteristic of an agent is the authority to make commitments for the principal to third parties. An exception might be under the theory of ostensible agency if the independent-contractor physicist worked with a patient under circumstances permitted by the principal that caused the patient to have reasonable belief that the physicist was an employee or agent and the patient relied on that belief. If the physicist gives guidance to dosimetrists, radiation therapists, nuclear medicine technologists, or radiology technologists, is he or she an independent contractor or an agent of the hospital upgrading the skills of hospital employees? Or, if the physicist implements a quality assurance program under the direction of the hospital Quality Assurance Committee, is this a non-delegable duty of that committee, which causes the consulting physicist to be an agent of that committee?

The status of a consulting physicist as either an independent contractor or as an agent will be determined at trial on the basis of the nature of the agreement under which the physicist worked, the activities of the physicist, and how the physicist functioned in the organization. If the physicist is found to be an independent contractor, neither the physician nor the hospital will generally be liable for the physicist's acts. However, the plaintiff may attempt to have the physician or the hospital or both at least share with the physicist in the liability for the physicist's negligent actions by showing faulty selection[75] or supervision of an independent contractor,[76] delegation of a nondelegable duty, or breach with respect to its own policies and rules.[77]

§ 18   Recommendations for Responsibilities of Medical Physicists from Reports Published by the American Association of Physicists in Medicine (AAPM)

In relation to diagnostic radiology, AAPM Report No. 33, dated April 1991, states:

> Physicists should direct and be responsible for the Quality Control (QC) programs. The foremost goal of these programs is to obtain and maintain optimal image quality and reliability while minimizing radiation exposure and ensuring compliance with radiation safety requirements. QC programs include diagnostic systems that produce or utilize ionizing radiation and other systems such as MRI and ultrasound that utilize non-ionizing radiations. A cost-effective practice is to designate a QC technologist to perform some of the measurements under the supervision of a physicist.[78]

AAPM Report No. 42, dated January 1994, states:

> While the imaging physician is responsible for the examination and fi-
> nal diagnosis, the medical physicist is responsible for the quality of the di-
> agnostic images, the safety (radiation, mechanical and electrical) of equip-
> ment, and the supervision of the techniques used by the technologist . . . .
> The medical physicist's first responsibility is to the patient and, conse-
> quently, there is an ethical obligation to seek outside reconciliation of the
> serious differences of opinion with regard to image quality and patient
> safety. [79]

Comment: These recommendations recognize that the physicist is qualified to supervise all of the steps required to produce quality images and
that placing the responsibility upon one person is operationally more effective than dividing the responsibilities among several people and can
lead to improved patient care and fewer lawsuits. Many suits have reached
the courts concerning missed or misinterpreted diagnoses on imaged fea-
tures in x-ray films, but the authors are aware of only one suit that has
been filed concerning the effectiveness of a mammographic imaging system. That suit was withdrawn by the plaintiff before it reached court. The
AAPM recommendation does not specify who should supply "reconciliation" regarding questions of image quality and patient safety. Infor-
mally, the mediator could be another member of the staff. More formally
the mediator may be someone with administrative authority.

In relation to radiotherapy, AAPM Report No. 38, dated 1993, states:

> The radiation oncologist holds the responsibility for verifying the diag-
> nosis and specifying the doses to be delivered to the treatment targets, as
> well as limitations on doses to critical structures. The physicist, however,
> should be aware of whether the prescription for a given patient is consis-
> tent with previous, similar patients, and also consider possible critical,
> dose-limiting structures. Any inconsistency noted by a physicist should
> be discussed with the radiation oncologist . . . .
>   While the radiation oncologist maintains the final responsibility for the
> patient's treatment, the physicist is responsible for the physical accuracy
> of the dose delivered. Thus, a physicist should not allow treatment to con-
> tinue until satisfied that all aspects of the treatment are sufficiently under
> control and that uncertainties in doses fall within acceptable tolerances. If
> any aspect of a treatment plan seems inappropriate to the point of being
> detrimental to the well-being of the patient or to the safety of the staff, and
> the radiation oncologist does not agree with such an assessment, the physi-
> cist has an ethical obligation to seek outside reconciliation of the differ-
> ence of opinion.[80]

Comment: Note the definition of two weighty responsibilities with legal
implications for the physicist. The physicist needs to be satisfied with *all*
aspects of the treatment relating to the physical accuracy of the doses delivered. This is equivalent to taking responsibility for the correct fulfillment

of the radiation dose prescription even though the physicist may not do all the steps involved. A related second responsibility is to challenge *any* aspect of the treatment that the physicist believes to be inappropriate, for example, a mistaken or misinterpreted prescription or radiation to healthy organs that exceeds that allowed by departmental policy. Again, the recommendation does not specify who should supply "outside reconciliation."

AAPM Report No. 46, published as Report of AAPM Radiation Therapy Committee Task Group 40, (April 1994) [81] states:

> The Joint Commission on Accreditation of Healthcare Organizations (JC-AHO) requires that quality assurance in radiation oncology be a part of the hospital's QA program (JCAHO, 1987)[82] and more recently, that a program of continuous quality improvement be implemented (JCAHO, 1992).[83] . . .
>
> . . . In order to assure the many facets of quality in the radiation oncology service, a Quality Assurance Committee (QAC) should represent the many disciplines within radiation oncology . . .
>
> . . . We recommend that the QAC oversee the QA program, have the responsibility of assisting the entire radiation oncology staff to tailor the recommendations of this and other reports to their radiation oncology practice, monitor and audit the QA program to assure that each component is being performed and documented, and write policies to assure the quality of patient care.
>
> *Radiation Oncology Physicist.* The radiation oncology physicist is responsible for the calibration of the therapy equipment, directs the determination of radiation dose distributions in patients undergoing treatment (i.e., computerized dosimetry planning or direct radiation measurement), and is responsible for the weekly review of the dose delivered to the patient. The radiation oncology physicist certifies that the treatment machine is performing according to specifications after it is installed, generates the data necessary for accurate treatment planning and delivery of the radiation therapy, outlines written QA procedures which include tests to be performed, tolerances, and frequency of the tests, and understands and appropriately responds to machine malfunctions and related safety issues. Moreover, the radiation oncology physicist should perform a yearly review of the policies and procedures manual of the department of radiation oncology . . . .[84]
>
> . . . Although a QA program for radiation therapy equipment is very much a team effort, and the responsibilities of performing various tasks may be divided among physicists, dosimetrists, and therapists, and accelerator engineers, we recommend that the overall responsibility for a machine QA program be assigned to one individual: the radiation oncology physicist.[85]

Comment: The 1994 AAPM Report No. 46 recommends that the radiation oncology physicist take "overall responsibility for a machine program," which requires less responsibility than "a physicist should not allow treatment to commence until satisfied that all aspects of the treatment are sufficiently under control," from the 1993 AAPM Report No. 38. Of course, if a quality control committee or administrative authority in a hospital assigns to the physicist responsibility for all aspects of quality assurance and the requirement to delay treatment until all aspects of the treatment are sufficiently under control, the functioning of the physicist would be the same under either recommendation. Probably, the lesser recommendation of 1994 reflects the policy or non-policy at most institutions in 1995. Some physicists may believe that their sole role is to perform certain technical duties. Other physicists may believe that they should have responsibility for the correctness of the fulfillment of the radiation prescription for each patient, which may be seen by dosimetrists, engineers, radiation therapists, or even radiation oncologists as an intrusion onto their turf. It would be interesting to know the fraction of radiation physicists who regard themselves as responsible for the correct fulfillment of radiation dose prescriptions. Informal inquiries by the authors suggest that a minority of radiation therapy physicists believe that they have this responsibility. If responsibility for the fulfillment of the radiation dose prescription is undefined or resides in several persons, the hospital or physician may retain responsibility as employer or, if the physicist is an independent contractor, as selector and supervisor of the physicist. Thus, there appears to be some uncertainty in the recommended responsibilities of radiation therapy physicists. Let us consider the responsibilities of nurses and pharmacists who have rather well defined roles, at least in traditional medical settings.

§ 19   Analogous Responsibilities of Nurses and Pharmacists

Both nurses[86] and pharmacists[87] have the following responsibilities and liabilities:

a. To fulfill correctly physician orders and prescriptions that the nurse or pharmacist knows will not harm the patient.
b. To *not* fulfill physician orders and prescriptions that the nurse or pharmacist knows may harm the patient. A discussion with the physician may resolve the issue of possible harm to the patient.[88] If the discussion does not settle concerns, the nurse or pharmacist should bring the difference of opinion to a higher administrative authority if that is possible and, if not, advise the physician to perform the procedure or deliver the prescription to the patient personally.[89]

Both nurses and pharmacists have relationships with patients in the absence of a physician. Medical physicists may also have relationships with patients in the absence of a physician; usually these are of a passive nature such as taking or being responsible for anatomical measurements of the patient or supervising the preparation of stabilizing molds. However, if the physicist is responsible for the fulfillment of radiation prescriptions, the legal positions of the medical physicist and the pharmacist are analogous; the two responsibilities listed above for pharmacists and nurses would probably apply to medical physicists.

As discussed above, in Lunsford v. Board of Nurse Examiners (1983),[90] the court held that the nurse's duty to a patient resulted from state licensure as a registered nurse in some cases. Probably most people who have a prescription filled rely upon the fact that the pharmacist is licensed by the state and believe that the pharmacist has a duty toward them. The effect of state licensure of medical physicists, where that exists, upon the duty of medical physicists to patients has yet to be developed.

§ 20   Questions and Provisional Answers on Responsibility

Who Is Responsible for the Integrity of Physical and Mathematical Systems in Radiation Oncology, Nuclear Medicine, Diagnostic Radiology, and Magnetic Resonance Imaging? Recommendations from the AAPM appear to place responsibility for the integrity of physical and mathematical systems in diagnosis and therapy upon the medical physicist. Unless there are written guidelines to the contrary at a particular institution, it would seem that responsibility for systems should reside with the medical physicist.

Who Is Responsible for the Quality of Diagnostic Images, Ensuring the Safety of Equipment, and the Supervision of the Techniques Used by the Technologists? Ensuring the quality of diagnostic images including supervision of techniques used by the technologists is the responsibility of the medical physicist, as defined by AAPM Report No. 42 quoted above.[91] Physicians who read diagnostic x rays, sonograms, and MRI images may define the desired quality of such images in various ways. Having physicists ensure that quality is a natural extension of their responsibility for the integrity of systems. However, there may be turf problems between physicists, physicians, and technologists.

Who Is Responsible for Verifying that a Radiation Prescription and Its Interpretation Are within Established Boundaries? Verification by the medical physicist that a radiation therapy prescription is within established boundaries is included in AAPM Report No. 38 but not in AAPM Report No. 46. This responsibility should be included in written guidelines or quality assurance procedures that have been validated by the hospital if the medical physicist is to be responsible for questioning a prescription as a pharmacist or a nurse would.

Who Is Responsible for the Correct Fulfillment of a Radiation Treatment Prescription? Responsibility by the medical physicist for the correct fulfillment of a radiation treatment prescription is included in AAPM Report No. 38 but not in AAPM Report No. 46 as stated above. The responsibility for the fulfillment of radiation treatment prescriptions includes more than ensuring the integrity of the machinery. It includes taking responsibility for the supervision of machine engineers, dosimetrists, and radiation therapists and for the many steps in prescription fulfillment. Again, whether a medical physicist is or is not to carry this responsibility should be documented in writing before the occurrence of a malpractice event. Later assignment of responsibility, after a malpractice claim has been made, is not satisfactory and is likely to be detrimental to the medical physicist.

Responsibility for the fulfillment of radiation therapy prescriptions should be considered from the perspective of what is best for the patient. A strong argument can be made that one person should be responsible for the entire complex chain of events from machine function and calibration to dose delivered, even though that person may not do the work. A poll of medical physicists would likely conclude that the medical physicist is the most qualified person or even the only person on site able to ensure the integrity of the entire chain of events in fulfilling a radiation therapy prescription. The allocation of responsibilities for the fulfillment of dose prescription is likely to differ at different facilities depending on the people involved, the degree of concern the hospital or radiation center has about malpractice, and, not least, the wishes of the medical physicist. All persons involved should unequivocally understand who is responsible for what. The opinion of the authors on this subject and the professional implications are given (in § 38).

5

REDUCING LIABILITY EXPOSURE

REDUCING THE PROBABILITY OF BEING SUED AND IMPROVING A DEFENSE IF SUED

§ 21   Quality Assurance Principles, Quality Assurance Guidelines, and Regulations

The quality assurance (QA) principles suggested below are meant to be broad, commonsense recommendations that support an attitude of continuing attention and of challenge to the correctness of medical use of radiation in diagnosis and therapy. They provide forethought to the possibility that actions of medical physicists may require legal defense. We distinguish *quality assurance principles* as general recommendations and *quality assurance guidelines* as specific actions relating to particular equipment and particular procedures. These categories are related and may overlap. References to some *published quality assurance guidelines* are made below.

A safety net of selective redundancies[92] is recommended to catch human errors or equipment malfunctions promptly and to increase the probability of managing a radiation misadministration successfully for the patient and the medical professionals concerned. Consulting physicists must pay particular attention to communication issues because they may not be present when unusual events occur. A shared basic attitude of open professional criticism, including challenges of one's own work, can go far in reducing barriers between professionals and building an effective safety net.

§ 22   Recommended Quality Assurance Principles—Organizational

The responsibilities and authority of various persons involved in applying radiation to patients can affect the quality of programs. Four thoughtful AAPM reports recommend organizational relationships and responsibilities of clinical medical physicists generally[93] in radiation oncology[94, 95] and in diagnostic radiology.[96]

In the following recommendations for quality assurance principles we use *shall* to mean mandatory actions, *should* to mean highly advisable actions, and *recommend* to mean advisable actions. The authors have no authority from any organization to require mandatory actions. We ask the reader to forgive our presumption so that we may use familiar terms for emphasis.

The organizational quality assurance principles recommended by the authors follow:

Principle 1. Responsibilities and authority of various persons involved with radiation medicine should be defined clearly.

Comment: Another defendant or even a plaintiff (as has happened) may try to define a physicist's responsibility retroactively from published recommendations.

Principle 2. Medical physicists should perform to national standards even though their employers may not expect it or do not allow them sufficient time to implement the standards.

Comment: A medical physicist cannot invoke overwork as an excuse for negligence; a professional should define the conditions for taking responsibility.

Principle 3. Supervisors should strive to develop an atmosphere of confidence and trust that encourages all persons involved to challenge procedures that they believe may harm a patient and to make their own errors known.

Comment: There is a legal basis for requiring both of these actions on the part of physicists (§ 36).

Principle 4. A physician should be designated to be informed about embryo or fetal irradiation and to counsel pregnant patients and pregnant radiation workers who have received or may receive radiation to the fetus.

Comment: Counseling requires knowledge[97, 98, 99, 100, 101] and sensitivity; a record of counseling should be kept.

Principle 5. Pertinent records should be retained for a period of time at least as long as the longest time possible in the statute of limitations for filing a cause of action for medical malpractice or for a period of time that other patient records are retained, whichever is longer.

Comment: Statute of limitations is discussed above (§ 10).

§ 23   Recommended Quality Assurance Principles—Radiation Oncology

A list of quality assurance principles for the practice of medical physics related to radiation oncology has evolved over a period of years that reflects insights gained from malpractice cases and other sources. Many of the principles are widely agreed upon; almost all of them could be important in the defense of a malpractice case. The quality assurance principles for radiation oncology we recommend are:

Principle 6. Appropriate redundancy shall be used to ensure that chamber calibration factors, atmospheric pressure corrections, wedge factors, transmission factors for each radiation shield, and other factors used in measurement and calculation are correct.

Comment: Radiation shields that appear the same may have different radiation transmission capabilities (particularly for low-energy electrons).

Principle 7. Radiation beams shall be calibrated with review by a second person at reasonable intervals, not to exceed one year. Output checks, which may be simply done, shall be made on therapy beams in order to call attention to a need for a calibration; daily checks on electrical machines and weekly checks on radionuclide units are recommended. For radionuclide units a comparison of measurements with predicted decay is recommended.

Comment: See examples (§§ 26, 27, 30). The weekly check of output of radionuclide units is recommended because there have been a number of instances in which teletherapy units have changed output with no external indication. For cobalt-60 teletherapy machines this change has happened when the source position is displaced mechanically in the "on" mode, when collimators have become broken but were still operative, or when source wheels have become unpinned from their axle. The one-week period between output checks allows a reasonable adjustment for patients undergoing treatment if the time of an output change is not known.

Principle 8. Independent checks of beam calibrations at an institution shall be performed on-site or by mailed dosimeters at reasonable intervals by individuals and equipment independent of the institution. It is recommended that mailed dosimeter checks be made at least quarterly.

Comment: Outside checks are important because an equipment fault or an error in calibration method is likely to be repeated without the error being revealed. See examples (§§ 28, 29). The quarterly recommendation comes from persons who offer such services. They note that an institution is more likely to irradiate the samples correctly on a quarterly basis than on a longer schedule.

Principle 9. Regular checks shall be made to ensure that machines are operated in the same way during calibration and during treatment. Quarterly checks are recommended.

Principle 10. The physical and electrical safety of patients undergoing treatment shall be reviewed at reasonable intervals. Quarterly checks are recommended.

Comment: Patients have been crushed by machine movement and injured by parts of machines or beam-defining accessories falling on them. Cardiac pacemakers may be affected by radiation producing machines.[102]

Principle 11. Only written radiation prescriptions shall be filled.

Principle 12. A posted or otherwise well-known departmental policy concerning the maximum radiation dose allowed to various healthy organs shall be observed in conventional treatments. If higher doses to healthy organs are intended, they shall be prescribed by the radiation oncologist.

Principle 13. A manual, calculated check of dose should be made to at least one point in each computer-generated treatment plan.

Comment: In some complex treatments a manual calculation may not be possible. In such instances accumulating a historical record on past patients may aid inexperienced persons in judging approximately the expected outcome of calculations.

Principle 14. An independent check of treatment plans shall be made by a second person.

Principle 15. For external beam treatments verification of machine settings by a second person acting independently or by passive monitoring of exposure time or monitor units by an automatic device shall be done.

Comment: Occasionally a patient has a very poor clinical result despite treatment records indicating no error. A contemporaneous check of the machine setting is strong evidence of correct machine use.

Principle 16. There shall be a weekly review of the accumulating patient dose in external-beam therapy.
  Comment: See example (§ 28).

Principle 17. Even minor changes in successful techniques shall be challenged for new hazards.
  Comment: See examples (§§ 32, 33).

Principle 18. The identity of the patient and the strength of brachytherapy sources or unsealed radionuclides used in radiation therapy shall be verified by a second person before fulfillment of a dose prescription.

Principle 19. Patients shall be surveyed with a radiation detector after removal of brachytherapy sources.

Principle 20. If an inconsistency is found in a treatment prescription, measurement, calculation, or functioning of a machine, that inconsistency shall be understood and resolved before proceeding with patient treatment.
  Comment: See examples (§§ 29, 30).

Principle 21. In the event of a misadministration of radiation treatment, the department head or a designee shall be informed promptly.
  Comment: Early bungling after a misadminstration can harm the patient and the legal posture of the health care providers.

Principle 22. Patient and physics records shall be protected, especially if a misadministration of radiation treatment has occurred.
  Comment: Participants in health care sometimes alter patient records. See example (§ 26).

Principle 23. Detailed records of the performance and maintenance of radiation machines shall be maintained.

Principle 24. Mechanical or electrical modifications of radiation machines shall be made only by the manufacturer or with the written approval of the manufacturer.

Principle 25. Malfunctioning radiation therapy machines shall not be repaired before a designated, responsible person is informed.
  Comment: See example (§ 30).

Principle 26. A malfunctioning radiation therapy machine or incorrect use of a machine shall not be repaired or corrected before the dosimetric consequences of the events are investigated and recorded.

Comment: See example (§ 30).

Principle 27. After any machine repair a radiation output check shall be made.

Principle 28. Before dosimetry methods are changed, the radiation oncologist shall be informed.

Comment: Physicians frequently compensate for dosimetry errors or idiosyncrasies in their treatment prescriptions.

A partial list of QA guidelines for radiation therapy is referenced.[103, 104, 105, 106, 107, 108, 109, 110, 111]

§ 24   Recommended Quality Assurance Principles—Nuclear Medicine

A few quality assurance principles of possible legal importance are recommended for physicists participating in nuclear medicine as follows:

Principle 29. Test the imaging capability of equipment by appropriate tests with comparison to recommended national standards. Tests should be performed daily or at a reasonable frequency to call attention to deteriorating imaging capability of equipment.

Comment: The integrity of a system should be such that the physicist can declare that the imaging capability of a particular machine on a particular day to a high degree of probability equaled or exceeded that required by a national standard of care. If no recognized standards exist for a procedure, the physicist should set reasonable internal standards until recognized standards appear.

Principle 30. Know and follow state or federal regulations and QA guidelines relating to licensing for ordering, possessing, testing, storing, labeling, posting warnings for, disposing of, and surveying for radioactive materials.

Principle 31. The suitability of radiopharmaceuticals, including radionuclide identity, quantity, quality, chemical purity, toxicity, sterility, and apyrogenicity, should be tested on site as far as that is possible. Those qualities of radiopharmaceuticals not tested on site should be reviewed in light of the provider's warranties and assurances.

Comment: At minimum the quantity of radioactive substances to be administered to a patient should be measured or verified on site. Equaling or exceeding the quality of practices in regard to pharmaceutical tests at similar installations, while not conclusive as an acceptable standard of care, is one of the considerations. See (§ 4).

Principle 32. Review of procedures for handling patients with therapeutic doses of radiopharmaceuticals should occur before each such event.

Comment: At many institutions therapeutic procedures do not occur often. Unpracticed procedures may present hazards to the patient, nurses, and radiation personnel.

A partial list of QA guidelines for nuclear medicine is referenced.[112, 113, 114, 115, 116, 117, 118]

§ 25   Recommended Quality Assurance Principles—Diagnostic Radiology, Ultrasound, and Magnetic Resonance Imaging

A few quality assurance principles of possible legal importance are recommended for physicists who participate in diagnostic radiology, ultrasound, or magnetic resonance imaging.

Principle 33. The imaging capability of equipment should be tested by appropriate tests with comparison to recommended national standards. Tests should be performed at a reasonable frequency to call attention to deteriorating imaging capability of a system.

Comment: The integrity of a system should be such that a physicist can declare the imaging capability of the system on a particular day to a high degree of probability equaled or exceeded that required by a national standard of care. If no recognized standards exist for a procedure, set reasonable internal standards until recognized standards appear.

Principle 34. Know and observe regulations and recommendations for limiting radiation to patients undergoing diagnostic radiology. For procedures that do not have guidelines keep radiation quantities as low as is reasonably consistent with imaging quality.

Principle 35. For a pregnant patient who has received radiation to the pelvic region measure or calculate the fetal dose and refer to Quality Assurance Principle 4 and its references.

A partial list of QA guidelines for diagnostic radiology is referenced.[119, 120, 121, 122, 123, 124, 125, 126, 127, 128]

6

SOME MALPRACTICE CASES INVOLVING MEDICAL PHYSICISTS

The malpractice cases described below are real events. In some instances details deemed extraneous have been omitted. For each example a physics comment and legal comment are given.

§ 26   Incorrect Decay of Cobalt-60 Source and Falsification of Records

Summary:

a. An incorrectly decayed cobalt-60 source resulted in increasingly more radiation than prescribed to patients over a period of 22 months ending at a 50% overdose.
b. Physicist falsified calibration documents.

Events: A cobalt-60 unit calibrated correctly initially was incorrectly decayed without remeasurement of the output. The fulfillment of patient radiation prescriptions increased progressively to 10% overdose in 5.5 months and then to 50% overdose in the subsequent 16.5 months. During the latter period 426 patients were treated. In 183 patients who survived beyond one year, there were 34% with severe complications in various sites including brain, spinal cord, skin, oropharyngeal mucosa, colon, and rectum.[129] Upon discovery of the patient overdoses, the institution notified the patients and referring physicians in those cases where the dose delivered to the patient was believed to be 10% or more than that prescribed. About 242 lawsuits were filed; all but one was settled out of court.

Initially the blame for the events was placed upon what was claimed to be a faulty measuring system. The physicist at the institution produced 10 calibration documents that supported the machine output used clinically during the 22 month period in question and stated that calibrations were not checked against the theoretical decay. The hospital notified the press of the radiation overdoses and of their belief that a faulty measuring instrument was the cause. Consultant physicists were called in to review the events shortly after the hospital had rectified the calibration error. When the consultants arrived, the ionization chamber that supposedly had been used for the 10 calibrations was found to be broken. The consultants established:

a. The cobalt unit was functioning correctly during the 22 month period in question. This conclusion was derived from the essential agreement between the initial calibration of the source and the calibration by the consultants with allowance for source decay.

b. The institution's ionization chamber and electrometer were operating correctly during the 22 month period in question. Orthovoltage x-ray calibrations and chamber comparisons performed with the same instrumentation during the same period were consistent with the proper functioning of the measurement instrumentation.

c. Five of the 10 calibration documents used atmospheric pressures that did not occur on the date stated. Retrospective atmospheric pressures were obtained from the National Climatic Center, Federal Building, Asheville, NC 28801.

d. The date on one chamber intercomparison document was changed between the first and second visit by the consultants.

e. Confronted with the above conclusions, the institution's physicist stated that all but one of the reported calibrations of the calibrations with the cobalt unit had not been done and that the calibration documentation had been generated without measurement.

Physics Comment: From the foregoing list of QA principles, calibration of the cobalt machine at reasonable intervals not to exceed one year, as recommended in Principle 7, would have been helpful. Mailed dosimeter checks, as recommended in Principle 8, would have revealed the problem sooner. A weekly check of machine output, as recommended in Principle 7, would have revealed the problem promptly. QA Principle 22 recommends protecting records. In this case, the medical physicist manufactured (falsified) records. Falsifying records is not a common event, but when it does happen it is likely to be discovered because of inconsistencies with other records. Falsified or lost records are damning in court. Comments and notations to records may be proper and legal if they are correctly identified and dated and there is no intent to misrepresent activities.

Legal Comment: Consider the elements of negligence. An ordinary, prudent physicist can calibrate a radiation therapy machine to within 2 to 3% of the calibration performed by another competent physicist with different instruments on the same machine. A court could easily find as the first element of negligence that the physicist had a duty to calibrate the cobalt-60 unit correctly by reason of his employment and that a national standard of care required calibration of a radiation therapy machine to within 3% or so. The physicist in this case had breached that duty (the second element of negligence). The third element of negligence concerns whether the patient sustained injuries as a result of the breach. Depending upon the dose prescription, arguments can be made to show that for treatment at many sites, patients can tolerate 15% or more radiation dose than that prescribed without injury and damage, but at other sites 15% overdose may not be tolerated. The fourth element of negligence, that there was damage to the patient, could be demonstrated easily for the patients who had received large overdoses (some had died from the radiation). Reference to textbooks or the literature is often helpful in deciding whether a higher (or lower) dose is likely to fall within the standard of care for a particular type of treatment. The defendants here assumed that all patients who had received overdoses of 10% or less had not been injured. They notified those patients (and their referring physicians) who had received more than a 10% overdose, inviting them to return for medical review. Legally this action had the effect of starting the clock on the statute of limitations. Over 240 cases were settled out of court. In the only case that went to court, the hospital stipulated that it was negligent in permitting 15% overdose and contested only the amount of damages. It is interesting that the plaintiff sued for $10 million, the institution had offered a settlement of $850,000, and the jury awarded $250,000.

§ 27   Miscalibration of Cobalt-60 Irradiator

Summary: A miscalibrated cobalt-60 replacement source resulted in a radiation dose 25% higher than prescribed.

Events: A replacement source in a cobalt-60 teletherapy machine was miscalibrated in such a way that the patients received 25% more radiation dose than prescribed. A factor of 0.8 was omitted in the denominator of the output calculations, perhaps reflecting an unrecorded shorter calibration-exposure time with the new source than was customary with the old source. The calibration of the new source was not checked by measurements of an independent person before being put into treatment service. Treatment of 207 patients occurred in the subsequent 5 months. During the latter half of that period the nursing staff noted unusually strong skin reactions in treated patients and communicated concerns to the physics staff. A review by the physics staff did not reveal the error. Presumably, the review was of existing records and did not involve new measurements. A routine review by an outside group that made new measurements revealed the error.

Physics Comment: Implementation of QA Principle 7 for weekly output checks likely would have revealed the calibration error unless the same data or calculation error was repeated. Check of beam calibrations on site by independent individuals (QA Principle 8) did in fact result in the discovery of the miscalibration.

Legal Comment: A calibration error of 25% would likely satisfy the first three elements of negligence (duty expressed in a standard of care, breach of duty, and injury due to that breach). Most medical physicists would agree that the standard of care would require a calibration within 2 to 3% of that regarded as correct. The 25% miscalibration was outside that standard of care, and the treated patients incurred some injury as a result of the miscalibration. However, the fourth element of negligence, damage, likely would have to be determined on a case-by-case basis. Depending upon the treatment site, some patients may have had long-term damage while others did not.

§ 28   Inadvertent Errors

Summary: Inadvertent or accidental errors do happen.

Events: Inadvertent errors are usually due to inattention and are distinguished from errors in which the person did what he or she intended but was wrong. Arithmetic mistakes, use of inapplicable data, faulty transfer of information, failure to include correction factors, or including correction factors more than once are examples of inadvertent errors. There is an unpublished study from a busy, major center in which a medical physicist reviewed five years of radiotherapy records in the 1970s. He found dozens or even hundreds of examples of inconsistencies that resulted in 10% to 35% more or less radiation delivered than prescribed. Prominent among the errors were bad math, misinterpretation of poor writing, data for one machine used for another machine, switching of digits in the final determination of machine setting, and use of an incorrect patient thickness for calculation. Not surprisingly, people with less experience were prone to making larger errors, but persons at all levels of experience made errors. Widespread inadvertent errors are confirmed in the experience of the Radiological Physics Center,[130] which reviews physics at institutions that participate in institutional clinical trials. Hundreds of errors of the types mentioned above were found in reviews of patient data from participating institutions, particularly in the 1970s. It is the impression of reviewing physicists that the incidence of inadvertent errors has declined in recent times. Perhaps the use of computers has reduced the number of such errors, particularly with software that makes explicit the treatment modality together with factors and patient parameters. However, the possibility of inadvertent errors still exists with the possibility of misunderstanding between humans or between humans and machines.

Physics Comment: QA Principle 14, an independent check of treatment plans by a second person, is practiced widely in the United States; the second person should be conscientiously independent. QA Principle 16, a weekly review of the accumulating patient dose in external-beam therapy, requires resources in time spent and yields a low return in errors discovered. However, an error discovered may avert a catastrophic result for a patient and the health care professionals. Clearly, if a retrospective review of five years of treatment can bring errors to light as discussed above, then a timely review that discovers errors while they are correctable is desirable.

Legal Comment: With certainty, physicists will be held to a standard of care that requires them not to cause injury because of inadvertent errors. It is no defense for a defendant to plead that the error is the only error made in thousands of opportunities. However, there is no system or program that can eliminate inadvertent errors completely. A medical physicist should ensure that reasonable safety nets are in place and due diligence practiced to discover inadvertent errors.

§ 29   Error in Atmospheric Pressure Determination and Choosing between Discrepant Alternatives

Summary:

a. Errors in obtaining atmospheric pressure necessary for calibrations that use ionization chambers open to the atmosphere may be due to miscommunication with weather stations or faulty use of aneroid barometers or both, sometimes confirming the error.
b. A radiation oncologist faced with differing calibrations of a cobalt-60 irradiator chose to continue with the older, incorrect calibration.

Events: Atmospheric pressure was incorrectly determined during cobalt-60 or linear accelerator calibration in four separate treatment centers by seven different physicists. Errors arose because physicists thought they were receiving station pressure from weather stations when in fact the pressures were corrected to sea level. Values for station pressure and pressure corrected to sea level are different; often weather station personnel do not clearly state which value is reported. A second type of pressure error resulted when traveling physicists from near sea level elevations made measurements at higher elevations and relied on a common type of aneroid barometer that had made a complete revolution and returned to scale. At altitudes of about 3,600 feet, both the weather station and the traveling barometer give about the same faulty pressure indication, which resulted in overdoses to the patient of 13% or 14%. In at least two of the treatment centers the same incorrect pressure was obtained redundantly by the two methods. At three of the centers, the overdose was 13%–14%, and at one center the overdose was 21%. In each instance many patients were treated.

The 21% overdose by a cobalt-60 teletherapy unit resulted from a faulty machine calibration that had been done with reliance upon an inquiry to a weather station for the atmospheric pressure. The atmospheric pressure obtained was corrected to sea level. The 21% overdose continued for 10 months until a different consulting physicist calibrated the machine and informed the radiation oncologist of the miscalibration. The radiation oncologist was faced with a 21% discrepancy between the two calibrations and chose to continue with the older, incorrect calibration. To our knowledge only two legal suits resulted, and these involved patients treated after the miscalibration was known. That the delivery of 21% more radiation than prescribed did not result in many lawsuits suggests that, at least at this institution, most patients could tolerate more radiation than prescribed. It is possible the radiation oncologist was compensating for the calibration error by lowering the dose prescription in some types of cases. In the two treatments that resulted in the filing of the legal actions, a nasopharynx treatment and a pelvic treatment, the patients apparently could not tolerate the additional radiation.

Physics Comment: Appropriate redundancy in determining atmospheric pressure as recommended in QA Principle 6 may have averted some of the miscalibrations. As recommended in QA Principle 8 (checking machine calibrations independently), mailed thermoluminescent dosimeters are not influenced by atmospheric pressure and were effective in calling attention to two of the miscalibrations. Implementing QA Principle 20 to understand the calibration discrepancy even at the cost of calling in a third physicist would have prevented the two overdoses in the 21% miscalibration.

Asking the weather station for both station pressure and pressure corrected to sea level would eliminate possible misunderstandings. Overall, calibration can be verified by mailed thermoluminescent dosimeters. In one of the instances of 13%–14% overdose due to the incorrect atmospheric pressure corrections, at a location with an elevation of about 3,600 feet, the institution regularly had the linear accelerator calibrated by consultants. One consultant relied on the misinterpreted pressure from the weather station. Another consultant's home base was near sea level, and the unrecognized full rotation of the barometer caused the same magnitude of error, confirming the erroneous calibration. The calibration discrepancy was discovered using mailed thermoluminescent dosimeters sent by the Radiological Physics Center (RPC). The RPC physicist sent to investigate the discrepancy made the same errors and agreed with the calibration in use at the hospital. The errors were faulty barometer reading and mistaken weather station pressure. During the visit brachytherapy sources were also measured with a portable ionization chamber that was open to the atmosphere.[131] The reviewing physicist for the RPC caught the problem by noting an apparent 13% discrepancy in the source strength of the brachytherapy sources between that stated by the source manufacturer and that measured by the portable chamber that required temperature-pressure corrections. Much closer agreement between the RPC measurements and the source manufacturer were usual. The reviewing physicist made a visit to the hospital and confirmed the calibration error of the linear accelerator as a result of the atmospheric pressure problem.

Legal Comment: Concerning the 21% overdose, at least two examples of negligence can be stated. A national standard of practice requires machine calibration to closer than 21%. The physicist did not adhere to the standard of practice in the calibration of the cobalt-60 unit, and patients were injured and sustained damage. The physician was also negligent. A court would almost certainly find that a national standard of care required a radiation oncologist to resolve a large inconsistency before proceeding with treatment, rather than choosing between discrepant alternatives. Atmospheric pressure may be measured or verified by mercury barometers, portable barometers, weather station inquiry, expectation at the elevation, and later reference to the National Climatic Center, Asheville, NC 28801.

In one of the incidents of 13%–14% overdose, patients sued for damages allegedly due to injuries resulting from overtreatment. The court held that the on-site physicist and the consulting physicists were not negligent. That four physicists independently had come to the same incorrect conclusion no doubt contributed to this verdict. Another possible contributing factor to the outcome is that 13%–14% overdose usually does not cause serious complications in patients. The physics community is likely to be divided about whether professional physicists are required to make correct measurements in the presence of misleading data. A different court might have reached a different conclusion.

The aftermath of discovery of the calibration problem in the same incident was managed well. The medical records of all 592 patients treated during the period of the machine miscalibration were reviewed by a panel of three radiation oncologists consisting of the radiation oncologist in charge and two outside consultants. The panel concluded that 75% of the patients were within the limits of the radiation dose prescribed by various practicing radiation oncologists for the conditions treated. Twenty-five percent of the patients received doses higher than those normally delivered for their conditions. Those patients deemed to have received more radiation than normally delivered were given special follow-up attention. All patients in both groups received written notification of the radiation overdose with a comment about whether their treatment was within or greater than normally delivered for their type of treatment. An invitation to discuss their situation further was included in the letter. This written notification (presumably with assurance that it was received by the proper person) has the legal effect of starting the clock on the statute of limitations in those jurisdictions in which the statute begins to run when the patient knew or should have known that an injury may have occurred (§ 10).

§ 30   Faulty Repair of a Linear Accelerator and Poor Communications

Summary:

a. A component failure in a linear accelerator was misrepaired, resulting in large overdoses in patient treatment.
b. The physicist was not informed of the component failure and repair.

Events: A linear accelerator capable of delivering a scanned electron beam of various energies between 7 and 40 MeV and an x-ray beam of 25 MV accelerates electrons in two fixed horizontal accelerator sections followed by two beam-bending magnets that cause the beam to change directions four times before entering the treatment head. In normal operation, in response to selection of a beam energy on the control panel, the equipment automatically controls the phase difference between the two accelerator sections, and thus, the energy to which electrons are accelerated, and also selects the appropriate current in the bending magnets for each beam energy to bring the beam to the treatment head. From time to time the power supply for the bending magnets failed in such a way that current to the bending magnets was for 32 MeV electrons regardless of the energy selected on the control panel. When that event occurred, the accelerator section continued to respond correctly to the lower energies selected, but the electrons did not reach the treatment head because of the mismatch between the energy of the electrons and the current in the bending magnets, except when an accelerator energy of 32 MeV was selected.

This failure in the power supply to the bending magnets occurred while a repairman from the manufacturer of the accelerator was in the area working on another machine. Instead of repairing the power supply to the bending magnets, he switched to manual control of the phase difference between the accelerator sections and caused the unit to operate at 32 MeV regardless of the beam energy selected. A meter on the control panel indicated that the beam energy was 36 MeV, but the machine operators initially assumed that this meter was in error. Neither the physicist nor the radiation oncologist were informed about the machine modifications and the modifications were not recorded in a maintenance book. Thus, persons who would have been familiar with the previous malfunctions and repair were not informed.

The machine was used in treatment for 10 days before the problem was recognized. At that time, the meter indication of 36 MeV was reported. Strong patient reactions to the radiation corroborated the existence of a problem. The malfunction and the patient treatments occurred between regular monthly check calibrations. Of 27 patients treated during this period for prescribed electron beams of 7, 10, or 13 MeV, 6 had died and 10 were hospitalized three months later.

Subsequent tests indicated that the patient doses were 7 to 10 times greater than those intended for 7-MeV electrons, 5 to 6 times greater for 10-MeV electrons and 3 to 4 times greater for 13-MeV electrons. These large factors may have arisen from the scanning function of the beam spreader operating at the lower selected energy, which resulted in the beam not filling the field, and, perhaps, not filling the monitor ionization chambers. What, if any, effect the malfunction had upon the x-ray beam is not known to the authors.

Physics Comment: There was not a system in place for notifying a responsible person of a malfunctioning radiation machine (QA Principle 25). An output check after a machine repair as recommended in QA Principle 27 likely would have revealed the problem before any patients were treated. QA Principle 7 recommends a daily output check on radiation beams. This can be done with a device such as a battery-operated solid state or ionization chamber detector, which can be placed at a fixed distance to integrate a short exposure. This simple check would have revealed the problem promptly. It is a very human response when something is broken or incorrect to fix it quickly and move on. However, in radiation therapy, the quick fix, as in this instance, may be incorrect, and if patients were treated while a machine was malfunctioning it is important to investigate what radiation dose those patients received (QA Principle 26). Often the malfunction cannot be recreated later.

Legal Comment: There are several examples of negligence in this event. The organization of the facility should have included firm rules concerning notification of a designated, responsible person when a radiation machine malfunction occurred and when a repair was made. A modern standard of practice would require that an employer designate such a person. The repairman from the accelerator manufacturer had some knowledge of the accelerator, but incorrectly held himself out to be an ordinary, competent repairman of this type of machine. His employer was culpable whether or not the employer had cleared the repairman to work on this type of machine since the repairman was functioning within the scope of his employment. The physicist who made only monthly output checks on the linear accelerator fell short of an acceptable standard of practice, which in most places consists of some kind of daily check (QA Principle 7).

§ 31   Design Error in a Linear Accelerator

Summary: An unorthodox manipulation of the controls of a linear accelerator resulted in a very high electron dose to two patients.

Events: A linear accelerator capable of treating with electrons and x rays used a computer to set and verify the various machine parameters after receiving an initial instruction for machine energy and for electron or x-ray mode. However, if an initial instruction for 25-MV x rays was changed to an electron beam instruction before the computer verification process for the first instruction was completed (about 20 seconds) the machine displayed the electron mode on the monitor in its usual format but operated partly from x-ray instructions and partly from electron instructions. Included instructions for x rays were high-beam current, 25-MeV energy, and no beam scanning; included instructions for electrons were for no target in the beam and for no x-ray beam flattener. This combination of operating parameters resulted in a high-beam current, unscanned 25-MeV electron beam with a diameter of about 5.5 cm at a depth of 2-3 cm. The machine recognized the high dose rate in the monitor chamber and turned the machine off within a second or so. However, in that short time 16,400 cGy was delivered by electrons at the depth of maximum dose. Measurements were made with thermoluminescent and ferrous sulfate dosimeters, both of which can be used at high dose rates. The results by the two measurement methods were in reasonable agreement, but attempts to measure with an ion chamber with correction for ion recombination were unsuccessful. The dose delivered was quite repeatable with a standard deviation for an individual observation of ±7% on replicate measurements.

The above chain of events that resulted in the machine setting the wrong parameters took place in the treatment of two patients. The first patient was being treated in the upper back area with 20 MeV electrons using a 10×17 cm^2 field. During a treatment in the second week the patient jumped up and said he felt as if he had received an electric shock and felt hot coffee poured on his back. The patient experienced vomiting, and later, paralysis in the legs and elsewhere. He died five months later. This account is not complete, but includes the elements required for discussion.

An exhaustive investigation by factory engineers and outside consultants did not reveal the problem. About three weeks later a second patient was being treated on the side of the face with 10-MeV electrons to a field of about 7×10 cm^2. The machine acted in the same manner as it had three weeks earlier. The patient said that he felt that he had been hit on the side of the face, saw a flash of light, and felt as though there had been fire on his face. The patient died three weeks later. After this event the physicist on site unraveled the chain of events and was able to reproduce the high dose experience by setting the machine for 25-MV x rays and then *quickly* changing the instruction to 10-MeV or 22-MeV electrons. The physicist called other radiation facilities that had the same type of accelerator. The same event could be reproduced on other machines.

Physics Comment: No practice of quality assurance would have uncovered this possibility of machine performance. A medical physicist at a radiation therapy installation would require extraordinary insight and confidence to challenge a manufacturer on the safety of an accelerator control system without an incident.

Legal Comment: In our view, the radiation professionals on site were not negligent in the event described. The manufacturer had a mechanism in place to turn the machine off that would function safely in almost all events involving excessively high dose rates. The physicist on site could not be expected to discover the design fault without a prompting incident. The fact that the fault was not discovered after the first event despite intense search by all concerned and outside consultants indicates the subtlety of the problem.

The legal theory of strict liability in products liability, however, would apply. The seller was engaged in selling such a product, the product was used without change in the condition in which it was sold, and the product was unreasonably dangerous to the user or consumer. It apparently had a design fault. Unreasonably dangerous is an objective standard to be judged by the ordinary prudent user of the machine.

Even though there seemingly was no way to protect the patient by a QA procedure in this instance, it is generally possible to help protect the medical professionals legally by QA procedures. Application of QA Principle 15 for verifying machine settings and monitor units as set could affirm the correctness or at least the apparent correctness of the machine settings. Mechanical, passive monitoring of machine settings for each treatment is persuasive in demonstrating correct machine use. However, if such capability exists on a machine but is not used, it is unfavorable to the defense of a malpractice suit.

§ 32   Small Technique Change Resulting in Injury to Patient (External Beam)

Summary: A long-established technique using cobalt-60 irradiators relied upon a generous cobalt-60 penumbra in matching the edges of fields. The penumbra was reduced when the technique was transferred to 8 MV x ray. The x-ray treatment resulted in over-irradiation of a small segment of the spinal cord with resultant paralysis of the patient.

Events: Treating neck nodes with a cobalt-60 beam to a supraclavicular field and to parallel opposed lateral fields to the neck was a textbook treatment. The edges of the anterior-posterior field and the lateral fields were matched on a line on the skin around the neck. With cobalt-60 treatment the spinal cord received about 4,700 cGy beneath the junction of the fields. When a similar treatment technique was used for the 8-MV x-ray machine, the dose to the spinal cord was estimated after the treatment to be greater than 5,500 cGy over a 2 mm segment of the spinal cord.

In the measurements and calculations, which were in remarkable agreement, the dose to the spinal cord could well have been higher due to a small geometrical uncertainties. Though there were other differences between the treatments with cobalt-60 and 8 MV x-ray treatment, we believe that the penumbra difference at the matching edges of the treatment fields was critical. The radiation treatment was intended to be prophylactic to nodes negative to cancer following the surgical removal of a malignant thyroid. The 11 year old patient became quadriplegic. The trial court awarded the patient over eight million dollars which was reduced to over five million (remittitur) by the appellate court.

Physics Comment: These events occurred in the mid-1970s when three dimensional calculations by computers were not available, but manual calculations to critical points could have been done. QA Principle 17 recommends investigating even minor changes in successful techniques for new hazards.

Legal Comment: The authors agree with the court judgment in the finding of negligence even though it is understandable how the events happened.

§ 33   Small Technique Change Resulting in Injury to Patient (Brachytherapy)

Summary: Gold-seed plaques for treatment of melanoma of the eye were well tolerated when the treatment was on the side or back of the eyeball but not on the front of the eye.

Events: A technique for treating melanoma of the eye with gold-seed plaques applied directly to the eye was used successfully with dozens of patients by a team of ophthalmologists and radiation oncologists. In most or perhaps all of these cases the tumor had been treated from the side or the back of the eye. The same technique when applied to a melanoma on the front of a patient's eye resulted in severe radiation destruction of the eyelid and rendered the eye orbit unable to accept an artificial eye.

The plaque conforming to the shape of the eye consisted of 15 gold-198 seeds configured with a central seed, an inner ring, and an outer ring. A lead shield 2.5 mm in thickness fit the spherical shape of the eye in providing shielding on the back side of the plaque away from the eye. The half-value thickness of lead for the gamma rays of gold-198 under broad beam conditions is about 3.3 mm. Allowing for curvature of the plaque and of the lead shield and considering the seeds individually, the dose to the eyelid opposite the center of the plaque was calculated to be 18,000 cGy. This high dose on the backside of the plaque when treatment was to the side or back of the eye apparently could be tolerated or at least resulted in damage that did not greatly interfere with the patient's life. On the front side of the eye the complications were serious.

Physics Comment: QA Principle 17 recommends investigating even minor changes in successful techniques for new hazards. If calculations on the back side of the plaque had been done, the dose of 18,000 cGy to the skin of the eyelid would have raised warnings.

Legal Comment: The case was settled out of court for a publicly undisclosed amount.

§ 34   Other Errors That Have Occurred

Some other types of physics errors that have occurred are listed here. Most of these events have not resulted in malpractice legal actions. This information is derived from many sources over a long period of time. For a quantitative expression of the effects of an incident we give the ratio of the radiation dose delivered to the patient, D, to the radiation dose prescribed, P, yielding a ratio of D/P.

Pancake Chamber Used Upside Down in Electron Beam Calibration:
Chamber was measuring at a greater depth than intended:

$$D/P = 1.20 \text{ for 6 MeV e}-$$
$$D/P = 1.10 \text{ for 9 MeV e}-$$
$$D/P = 1.08 \text{ for 12 MeV e}-$$
$$D/P = 1.00 \text{ for 16 MeV e}-$$
$$D/P = 0.99 \text{ for 20 MeV e}-$$

Calibration Errors and Clinical Compensation: Three hospitals were served by the same group of three radiation oncologists and two physicists. The radiation therapy calibrations at the three hospitals resulted in $D/P = 1.08$, $D/P = 1.00$, and $D/P = 0.92$, due in part to different calibration equipment at each place. Remarkably, the same radiation oncologist gave different dose prescriptions at different hospitals for similar treatments, compensating for the calibration errors.

Error in Table Lookup Using TG-21 Protocol: Two physicists at different institutions made the same error in looking up the mean restricted collision mass stopping power ratio for calibration of 18 MV x rays and 20 MV x rays using the TG-21 protocol. In each instance the value interpolated by the physicist from the protocol was 1.101, but the value used was 1.011.

$$D/P = 1.09 \text{ (2 institutions)}$$

Inverse Square Correction for Lesser or Greater Treatment Distance Included in Computer Program and Also Applied Manually:

$$D/P = 0.79 \text{ (institution A)}$$
$$D/P = 1.56 \text{ (institution B)}$$
$$D/P = 0.88 \text{ (institution C)}$$

Treatment on Source Axis Distance (SAD) System But Dosimetry Calculated on Source Skin Distance (SSD) System:

$$D/P = 1.16$$

Incorrect Depth Dose Data Used to Calculate D-max from Calibration Position at 5 cm: Four MV x-ray data was used instead of 10-MV x-ray data.

$$D/P = 0.90$$

Ionization Chamber Partly Shielded during Measurements of Asymmetric Fields: Chamber remained on machine central axis during measurements with collimators in asymmetric positions.

$$D/P = 1.06 \text{ to } 1.30$$

Dose to Each of Two Fields Confused with Intended Total Dose at Intersection of Central Rays:

$$D/P = 1.68 \text{ (institution A)}$$
$$D/P = ? \text{ (institution B–award to plaintiff)}$$

Data Entered into Computer Incorrectly: Prior depth dose entries were erased with new entries. For all fields below 20 x 20 cm^2 the computer extrapolated the data.

$$D/P = \text{up to } 0.90$$

Faulty Extrapolation of Measured Data: Computer program used zero as percentage depth dose beyond 25 cm depth. A very large patient was overtreated.

$$D/P = ?$$

Wedge Used in Treatment but Wedge Transmission Factor Was Not Included in Calculation:

$$D/P = 0.81 \text{ (institution A)}$$
$$D/P = 0.80 \text{ (institution B)}$$

Wedge Transmission Factor Used in Calculations but Wedge Not Used in Treatment:

$$D/P = 1.24 \text{ (institution A)}$$
$$D/P = 1.11 \text{ (institution B)}$$
$$D/P = 1.15 \text{ (institution C)}$$
$$D/P = 1.41 \text{ (institution D)}$$

Wedge Transmission Factor Entered Twice: A wedge transmission factor was entered in calculations two times, redundantly.

$$D/P = 1.53 \text{ (institution A)}$$
$$D/P = 1.22 \text{ (on boost only; institution A)}$$
$$D/P = 1.25 \text{ (institution B)}$$

Two Fields Treated but Calculations Were for Three Fields:

$$D/P = 0.60$$

Confusion of Dose to a Selected Isodose Level and Dose to Isocenter or to Other Isodose Line:

$$D/P = 1.11 \text{ (4 institutions)}$$
$$D/P = 1.15 \text{ (1 institution)}$$
$$D/P = 1.20 \text{ (1 institution)}$$

Treatment Was with 18 MV X Ray but Calculations Were for 6 MV X Ray:

$$D/P = 1.17$$

Air Gap Correction Not Included in Electron Beam Calculation:

$$D/P = 0.83$$

A New Cesium Brachytherapy Source Contained No Radioactivity
Source was not used in treatment.

Incorrect Point "A" Location in Pelvic Brachytherapy:

$$D/P = 0.55 \text{ (institution A)}$$
$$D/P = 0.66 \text{ (institution B)}$$

§ 35   A Medical Physicist Encounters the Law (3) (Story continued from § 16)

Pretrial discovery procedures by the plaintiff included the production of things, particularly all the medical records of the plaintiff, including copies of physics calculations relating to the case. By this time both the plaintiff and defendants had engaged a radiation oncology expert and a physics expert. The plaintiff submitted written interrogatories to the defendants based upon the medical records he received; written interrogatories are very specific questions that require a written answer under oath from the other party, in this case, the defendants. The defendant obtained an order from the court, without objection from the plaintiff, to obtain medical records pertaining to the treatment of skin malignancies on the face of the plaintiff by other medical entities before the time the plaintiff entered treatment by the defendants. Medical reviews of the plaintiff's eye subsequent to the radiation treatment were also requested.

The radiation oncologist, the physicist, and one of the radiation therapists separately gave depositions under oath. The lawyer for the plaintiff questioned them about the adequacy of their training, their experience, their usual duties, and the events of this case. The lawyer for the defendants made objections to some of the questions. These objections were noted by the court reporter in the record of the deposition. The lawyer for the defendants also asked questions that led to answers favorable to the defense.

DR. THOMAS T. BREWSTER, M.D.

In deposition Dr. Brewster stated:

1. *Treatment of eyelids by low-energy electrons commenced over 25 years earlier at some major centers and is well documented. Further, he stated that he had made an extended visit to a major center to learn the technique and followed that technique in his practice. He also used low-energy x rays to treat some skin lesions.*
2. *Prior to treatment, the patient was informed that the tear glands might be destroyed in the proposed treatments. The patient gave his consent to proceed.*
3. *Physicist, Barbara Hickman, had reviewed the treatment proposed for the plaintiff, Marvin G. Stifler, prior to the treatment. She recommended the electron beam modality rather than low-energy x rays because the squamous cell carcinoma in the left eyelid extended well into the left eyebrow above the bone of the supraorbital arch. She made the point that with electrons the energy absorption in bone is about the same as in skin but with the low-energy x rays the energy absorption in bone could be two to four times greater than in skin depending upon the energy and filtration of the x ray. The electron treatment would be well tolerated by the bone, but the x-ray treatment might result in permanent damage to the bone.*
4. *When Ms. Hickman was hired she asked that she have the responsibility and the authority to ensure that radiation dose prescriptions were fulfilled properly. Dr. Brewster stated that he agreed, although somewhat reluctantly.*

BARBARA M. HICKMAN, M.S.

In deposition Ms. Hickman stated:

1. *By agreement she was responsible for the fulfillment of the radiation treatment prescriptions at Mountain View Cancer Center.*
2. *She followed published recommendations for care of radiation measuring instruments by instrument calibration every two years and monthly constancy checks in a commercial chamber checker.*
3. *The calibration of various radiation beams followed published protocols.*
4. *On the linear accelerator, the radiation therapists measured all beams each treatment day with an easily-used device with a solid state detector. If readings differed by more than 3% from that expected, Ms. Hickman was notified. Ms. Hickman compared the solid state detector to the calibration chambers regularly. All measurements were recorded in bound books.*
5. *Quarterly Ms. Hickman received mailed thermoluminescent dosimeters from an independent laboratory, irradiated dosimeters with each beam, and mailed the irradiated dosimeters back for analysis and for comparison with her statement of dose. These independent measurement results were within acceptable agreement with calibrations she was using for 6 MeV electrons before and after the treatments of the plaintiff.*
6. *Ms. Hickman stated that the calibration of her instruments and check of her machine calibrations by outside independent entities together with daily beam measurements and other constancy checks meant that the radiation in the electron beam used for treatment of the plaintiff was consistent from day to day during the therapy and was in agreement with national radiation standards.*
7. *Ms. Hickman stated that on one day during the period of treatment of the plaintiff she was notified by the radiation therapist that the linear accelerator was stopping abruptly during treatment and required several machine restarts to complete a treatment. Ms. Hickman directed that the treatments be stopped. She verified by measurement that the machine delivered the expected amount of radiation despite the interruptions of the beam. She called the accelerator maintenance firm; they suggested making an adjustment, which she did. The beam interruption problem ended. She remeasured the beams assuring that the calibrations had not been altered by the adjustment. All of these activities were recorded in a bound book.*
8. *Ms. Hickman stated that the linear accelerator did not have an electromechanical device for verifying the machine settings for each*

treatment. However, one of the two radiotherapists assigned to each machine set the machine parameters, and the second radiotherapist conscientiously and independently verified the settings for each treatment. Both initialed the record for each patient each treatment day. Ms. Hickman checked the integrity of the process at least each month.

9. *Ms. Hickman stated that she can state with a high degree of confidence that the prescribed dose was delivered in the treatment of patient, Marvin G. Stifler.*

10. *Ms. Hickman acknowledged that the eye shield used in Mr. Stifler's treatment apparently had been thrown out by a cleaning person after Mr. Stifler's treatments but before he initiated a lawsuit. She had measured the transmission of 6 MeV electrons through one of the identically appearing eyeshields but did not know if that eyeshield were used in the treatments of Mr. Stifler.*

The experts on both sides made measurements to determine the radiation dose to the cornea (surface) and lens (0.5 cm-depth) of the plaintiff's left eye. In these measurements the expert for the defense had a considerable advantage in using a measurement situation closely simulating the treatment of the patient. Measurements were with 6-MeV electrons directed frontally to the eye with the same machine that was used in treatment. An irregular cutout block to limit the area of the treatment was refabricated from notes in the patient records. Six layers of 1.5-mm dental wax was used as bolus to ensure full electron buildup on the eyelid as in the treatment. The transmission through the lost eyeshield was uncertain. The transmission of one of the identical-looking eyeshields had been measured before the plaintiff's treatment. The defendant's physics expert was dismayed to find that the electron transmission through the eyeshields of the same type and manufacture differed by as much as a factor of two even though the shields appeared to be identical. Because the eyeshield used in treatment had been lost, the best that could be done was to take an average and a maximum of the transmission of six similar eyeshields that had been collected. Through this procedure the expert witness demonstrated that either the average or the maximum transmissions through the eyeshields that were measured would have resulted in a dose to the cornea and to the lens of the patient's eye that was less than the dose regarded as tolerable in the literature.

(This story is concluded in § 44.)

7

WHEN THINGS GO WRONG

§ 36 In Normal Operations—Responsibilities between Employer and Employee, Errors, and Ownership of Records

Employer Responsibility to Employee; Employee Responsibility to Employer: There is a well-established legal doctrine called *Respondeat Superior,* which means "let the master answer." Under this doctrine, the wrongful acts of an employee in the course of his or her employment are the responsibility of the employer. The doctrine is not applicable when the employee is acting outside the legitimate scope of his or her employment. A physicist who is an employee of a hospital but who consults privately to another institution is acting outside the scope of his or her employment by the hospital. The employing hospital is not responsible for the physicist's acts at another hospital.

An employee has a responsibility to minimize liability to his or her employer. A physicist is responsible for the correctness and safety of those activities within his or her areas of responsibility; there is also a general obligation to call attention to other hazards for which the physicist may not have direct responsibility.

Prevent Harm to a Patient: A medical physicist, similar to a nurse or pharmacist, has a responsibility to call attention to anything, including orders of physicians, that may harm a patient (§ 19). If a dispute with a prescribing or ordering physician cannot be resolved, a physicist may be obligated to take the question to a higher authority. The physicist should strive to create an atmosphere in which he or she can provide input to the medical decision process. However, the physician is responsible for medical decisions. Today, direct challenges to physicians' medical decisions without compelling reasons based on medical physics are taken only with some professional risk to the physicist. If there is no higher authority, the physicist may provide some self-protection by putting the concerns in writing to the physician. Writing these concerns directly on a patient's chart is generally not proper because those notes can undermine the radiation therapy team and provide no benefit to the patient.

A few years ago when one of us (RJS) was chairman of the American Association of Physicists in Medicine Ethics Committee, the committee had a question of what to do from a medical physicist who had tried unsuccessfully to dissuade a radiation oncologist from a planned procedure. The quick answer seemed easy: put your recommendations in writing to the radiation oncologist and abide by his decision. However, a 1965 Illinois case, Darling v. Charleston Community Memorial Hospital,[132] may indicate a different answer here. In that case a physician who was not an orthopedic specialist set a broken leg while on duty in the emergency room. The hospital did not have a specialist review the case nor did the hospital-employed nurse report that the patient was showing blue toes. The patient lost the leg because the cast constricted the blood supply to the leg. For the first time, a hospital and its board were held responsible for the quality of a physician's performance. This decision implied hospital responsibility greater than ensuring that doctors practicing in the hospital were properly licensed and in good standing with the appropriate medical societies.

The more considered answer to the above question is that a physicist should discuss the planned procedure with the physician; if the physician continues in the treatment, the physicist has a duty to protect his employer from liability by informing the appropriate person. If the physician is the employer, the recommendation to change treatment should be made in writing to the physician. If the hospital is the physicist's employer, the physicist should advise the appropriate administrator to review the case.

Several lawyers who specialize in medical malpractice concur with the view that a physicist has a responsibility to protect his or her employers from liability if the physicist thinks that a medical mistake is about to be made, despite the risk of losing cordial relations with a physician.

Legal Need for Revealing Own Errors: Many medical physicists have discovered their own errors. The error may relate to a patient under treatment and be therefore correctable or may be a systematic error that has affected previous patients. What is the physicist's ethical and legal responsibility?

Radiation therapy is still an empirical art. For various types of treatment, the correlation between radiation dose and clinical responses is crucial in the skillful use of this modality. If the determination of radiation dose is unreliable for whatever reason, the radiation oncologist may be severely handicapped in decisions on dose prescriptions. If the medical physicist is unwilling to reveal past physics errors, the skill of the radiation oncologist may be undermined in treating new patients because of a faulty association of dose prescriptions and the expected clinical result. The temptation of a physicist to correct physics errors without bringing those errors to clinical attention could result in future patients receiving more or less treatment than optimum within the experience of the radiation oncologist. Clearly the medical physicist is under an ethical obligation to reveal his or her own or another's errors. It is reasonable to have an agreement with those concerned that errors of less than a certain amount, say 2%, be corrected without notification and documentation.

Legal theories under a broad category of misrepresentation and nondisclosure may be applicable by a radiation oncologist against a physicist who conceals errors. Deceit is a long-identified tort of misrepresentation.

> The elements of actionable deceit are: a false representation of a material fact made with knowledge of its falsity, or recklessly, or without reasonable grounds for believing its truth, and with intent to induce reliance thereon, on which plaintiff justifiably relies to his injury.[133]

Turning back the odometer of a used car has been held to be deceit.

> Again, one who has made a statement, and subsequently acquires new information which makes it untrue or misleading, must disclose such information to anyone whom he knows to be still acting on the basis of the original statement—as, for example, where there is a serious decline in the profits of a business pending its sale.[134]
>
> ... there has been a rather amorphous tendency on the part of most courts in recent years to find a duty of disclosure when the circumstances are such that the failure to disclose would violate a standard requiring conformity to what the ordinary ethical person would have disclosed. The issue has been regarded as one for the court rather than the jury.[135]

Most of the legal theory relating to deceit has come from commercial contexts such as contracts and sales. Deceit can be shown if the defendant knows or believes that his or her representations are false or have insufficient basis in fact and that the defendant has the intention to induce the plaintiff to rely upon the misrepresentations resulting in the plaintiff's injury and damage. Fraud and deceit have the same elements and usually involve ways in which another person is cheated. The authors are aware of instances in which they believe medical physicists have corrected their errors and deliberately withheld that information from clinicians in order to preserve their reputations and perhaps employment. It is not clear that this degree of deception would rise to the level of the intentional tort of fraud. However, there can be little doubt that the act of withholding knowledge of a significant change in radiation dose delivery would at least be negligent misrepresentation or negligence. Lawyers, accountants, and other professionals, in order to avoid professional negligence, are often expected to correct statements to clients that the professional later finds to be untrue.

Ownership of Records: A physicist who is an employee is paid to make radiation measurements. Records of measurements are part of the physicist's work product, and those records are the property of the employer. The employer has a legal duty to maintain them as patient care records. When a physicist leaves his or her employment, he or she sometimes takes all or some of the records without permission. Such an action is wrong and, in some cases, may constitute theft. When a departing physicist wishes to take computer programs or systems he or she has devised, a satisfactory agreement can usually be made with the employer giving permission for the physicist to copy the requested records.

The removal of physics records can leave an incoming physicist and the institution in a crippled position clinically and legally with regard to previously treated patients. Vigorous actions, including the pressing of criminal theft charges against a departing physicist by an institution, are justified to prevent loss of physics records.

The other side of this issue relates to assigning responsibility for the correctness of data and systems that a physicist leaves in place after departing employment. The new physicist should verify and stand behind measurements, calculations, and systems; the departing physicist cannot be responsible for how a system is used or misused. A simple release of responsibility from the employer to the departing physicist can be written by any lawyer.

§ 37   When a Patient May Have Been Injured

Investigate Incident before Making Corrections: A malfunctioning radiation therapy machine may change its output or produce a distorted radiation beam. Measurements of the malfunctioning machine and an estimate of when the malfunction started are necessary to understand the dose pattern delivered to patients under treatment and to plan compensatory modifications to treatment. Sometimes the malfunction cannot be recreated. See Quality Assurance Principle 26.

Preserve Records after an Incident: It is uncommon for records to be altered or destroyed by physicians, physicists, or hospital employees who wish to protect themselves, but it does happen. Efforts to alter or destroy records usually harm the defendant's case. The integrity of records should be ensured by copying or other precautions.

Notification of Insurance Company: Insurance policies will include procedures for notification of the carrier when an insured incident occurs. Failure to notify the carrier properly could result in loss of insurance protection for the incident.

Notification of Regulatory Agencies: State or federal regulations may require some special notifications and record keeping for radiation dose administrations that differ from those prescribed by the radiation oncologist. Reports of a *recordable event* must be retained at the institution for review by regulatory inspectors. *Misadministrations* are *reportable* to the regulatory agency. In federal regulations[136, 137] for cobalt-60 irradiators (and x-ray machines under some state regulations), a recordable event occurs if the weekly dose to a patient exceeds 15% of that intended. A misadministration occurs if the weekly dose to a patient exceeds 30% of that intended or the total dose exceeds 20%. For brachytherapy, the criteria for the difference of dose delivered and that prescribed for a recordable event is 10% and for a reportable misadministration is 20%. Notification of a misadministration to both the referring physician and the patient is mandatory for misadministrations and discretionary for recordable events.

A radiation oncologist who notifies a patient of a misadministration could distinguish between the requirements of the regulation and the complications, if any, to be expected by the patient on the basis of scientific and medical evaluation of the particular case.

Engage a Personal Lawyer: Today it is unlikely that a medical physicist will get through his or her professional career without needing an attorney. Contract law, employment law, and personal injury law present too many occasions that require advice of counsel. Medical physicists may want to develop a relationship with an attorney much like one does with a family physician. A personal attorney can assist the medical physicist in matters that come up from time to time and will be in a position to recommend other counsel when a legal specialist is needed.

A medical physicist loses significant control over his or her destiny when sued. The physicist may not even have a choice of the attorney who will prepare the primary defense of his or her case. Attorneys may be appointed by the insurance company if the physicist possesses malpractice insurance. Though it is against the law, attorneys occasionally put the interest of the insurance company above that of the client. A physicist should be sensitive to this possibility and raise objections to both the attorney and the insurance company if his or her interests are not being properly addressed.

Joint representation of defendants in lawsuits is another common practice that physicists should view with caution. For example, defendant physicians, physicists, and institutions may be insured by the same company; this company may assign a single law firm to represent several or all of the defendants. Often the legal defenses and interests of the various defendants are significantly different and cannot be properly represented by a single attorney or law firm. A personal attorney can be of help in this situation. Even if the physicist's attorney does not conduct the defense, that attorney can follow the case and look after the physicist's interests. A prior understanding about the level of participation of the physicist's attorney and the legal fees is recommended.

What to Tell the Patient: It is not the physicist's task to decide what to tell a patient or the referring physician when a mistake has been made, but the physicist may advise. A correct but unspecific answer is to tell the patient that which would be told by an ordinary, prudent physician under the same circumstances. Reference to textbooks and the periodical literature to establish background knowledge may be very important to a patient who has received more radiation than actually prescribed but not more radiation than routinely prescribed elsewhere for similar treatment. It is important that the patient be made aware of medical complications that may result from the mistake and be advised of ways of coping with the complications. A patient is less likely to sue if he or she is not charged for extra medical attention.

Start the Clock on the Statute of Limitations: States will differ in the amount of time after an event within which a lawsuit must be filed and in the manner of initiating the statutory period. In some states the period is two years after the patient knows or should have known of a mistake. A lawyer should advise possible defendants (§ 10).

Answering Questions: Questions should be answered truthfully, directly, and briefly. It is not appropriate, generally, to volunteer information not germane to a question or to answer questions not asked.

8

EDITORIAL AND PROFESSIONAL VIEWS

§ 38   Responsibilities for Correct Fulfillment of Dose Prescription

In most radiotherapy installations, the physicist is the only person who can trace the entire chain of events from the care of measuring instruments through machine or source calibration and radiation distributions to a statement of dose delivered to a patient. Because in fact this responsibility rests directly or indirectly upon the physicist, the physicist should openly take credit or blame for the correctness of dose fulfillment. The importance of this function in effective therapy and in avoiding malpractice lawsuits should be made clear to management. Taking responsibility is the mark of a professional, as opposed to a technician, who may do complex functions but often does not take responsibility for the result. A professional who accepts responsibility does not have an excuse for not fulfilling that responsibility. Overwork or lack of equipment are not excuses for failure to uphold a responsibility. A professional should define the conditions under which he or she will accept responsibility. The earnings of a professional are more related to the responsibilities taken than to the hours worked and the technical complexity of that work.

§ 39   "Proof" That a Radiation Prescription Has Been Fulfilled Correctly

Sometimes a patient has a response to radiation treatment that is consistent with radiation overdose but all the radiotherapy and physics records indicate that no overdose has occurred. There might be some question or even general evidence that the physicist had not done his or her work correctly. The physicist could be in a position of needing to prove that the dose prescription was correctly fulfilled. "To prove" here is in the legal sense of a civil suit and means to prove that something is more probable than not. Leading a jury through a calibration protocol is a daunting if not impossible task that would still leave open the possibility of incorrectly recorded data. However, an independent verification of machine calibration at a time before and after the treatment with a demonstration of machine consistency during the period between the independent verifications as recommended in QA Principles 7 and 8 is readily accepted. Independent evidence that the machine was set correctly as recommended in QA Principle 15 likely will be accepted because it is a positive, contemporaneous record. Finally, a demonstration of correct machine performance by regular output checks as recommended in QA Principle 7 and by keeping adequate maintenance records as in QA Principle 23 is likely to be persuasive. This type of data together with calculations relating to the patient should make a case that it is more probable than not that a radiation prescription was fulfilled correctly.

§ 40   Government Regulations—Reporting Misadministrations

When the aim of governmental regulators is the reasonable radiation protection of the radiation user and others nearby, the regulators perform an important function. However, when regulators try to regulate functions that are close to the practice of medicine and medical physics they have the same goal as the medical professionals—the effective and safe delivery of radiation to patients in diagnosis or treatment. In that endeavor, the medical professionals have vastly greater training and experience than the regulators can possibly have. The careers of the medical professionals depend on the effective and safe use of radiation.

A reportable misadministration of treatment may or may not have medical consequences for the patient. The forced reporting, notification of the patient, and publication of the misadministration by the regulatory agency may result in alarming a patient unnecessarily. Some physicians in some instances would take the position that notification is likely to harm the patient. This might be the case if the radiation dose exceeded the prescription sufficiently for reporting but was still within commonly accepted boundaries. If a physicist is the radiation safety officer (RSO) responsible for reporting the misadministration, the physicist has no option but to report to the regulatory agency, whatever the consequences to the patient, the institution, and relationships between the medical professionals. A physicist who is also the RSO may be brought into conflict with a radiation oncologist who does not want to report a misadministration.

In notification of the patient, as required by regulations, the physician can evaluate the possible harm to the patient, possible complications, and make an offer of free further treatment if that becomes necessary. If the physician believes that in this particular instance there is no or small consequence to the patient, that can be fully explained to the patient together with a statement that patient notification is a required formality. Of course, there may be retribution visited upon the physician by the hospital management or the liability insurance company in response to the publication of the misadministration by the regulatory agency.

A physicist who is also the RSO and who is repeatedly placed in irreconcilable controversy with the radiation oncologist over reporting of misadministrations could sidestep the issue by recommending that the radiation oncologist become the RSO with responsibility for reporting and the physicist become an assistant. Probably, a better solution is to involve a hospital committee in the process, perhaps a Quality Assurance Committee. Possibly some state regulatory agencies would grant authority to a responsible committee to decide upon the notification of patients in particular cases. Even if regulatory agencies do not give that permission, involving the hospital administration early in a reportable event may diminish the severity of the hospital's response toward their own staff that may result from the actions of the regulatory agency.

It may be too soon to judge the usefulness of the reporting regulations relating to radiation therapy. The early response of physicists is often to begrudge the time and effort to cope with the regulations and to separate the regulations from the functional QA system.

§ 41 Regulations Should Not Be Used as a Weapon

In the last nearly 100 years the collaboration between radiation oncologists and physicists has been hugely effective in developing radiation therapy as a reliable treatment for cancer. That success has resulted in the growth and the professional well being of both professions. In recent years, radiation oncologists have attracted patients to an institution with their skill and reputation and thus have acquired power in the medical area. With the turmoil now occurring in the organization of medicine in the move toward managed care, administrators are becoming more important in bringing patients to a hospital than physicians. Thus, the political clout of administrators is increasing and that of physicians is decreasing. Predictably, this change of relative status between radiation oncologists and administrators will not be gentle, particularly for experienced physicians. Physicists may well find that their relative status will improve in the transition to managed medical care. The editorial advice offered here to physicists is to remember that the success of radiation oncology has resulted from the creative collaboration between physicist and physician and that a productive relationship between them is to the benefit of the patient, physician, and physicist. A temptation to use radiation regulations against the radiation oncologist by the physicist RSO has been seen in at least two instances by the authors. Administrators may even encourage physicists in this activity in order to enhance their own posture and diminish that of radiation oncologists. We here urge physicists not to play this game.

§ 42   Protection of Assets

Some physicians, lawyers, and medical physicists protect their personal assets and do business without liability insurance protection. The logic flows from the belief that plaintiffs will be discouraged from suing a defendant without significant available assets. More conventionally, professionals have liability insurance that pays legal defense costs and also damages against the professional up to specified limits. Thus, lawsuits without merit are defended without cost to the insured, and meritorious cases are tried or settled with the possibility of justice to the plaintiff without bankrupting the defendant.

A prudent position for a professional may be a combination of liability insurance, purchased by the professional's employer, by the professional, or both, and protection of the professional's most important personal assets. Asset protection may take the form of limited partnerships, limited liability companies, corporations, and trusts. All of these require money and time to establish and also continuing effort. All partners in a conventional partnership are liable for the actions of one partner. Limited liability partnerships are possible. A professional will want to weigh his or her exposure to liability against the need to protect personal assets.

Protection of assets and estate planning is a legal specialty available in urban areas. Some of these legal specialists give seminars, particularly to physicians. Medical physicists can find out about these seminars by asking physicians if they have received any advertising on this topic. One of us (RJS) has attended seminars by a national firm[138] as well as seminars offered by local legal firms.

An attendee at a local or national seminar can gain sufficient information to judge whether he or she needs or wants asset protection. If an attendee decides to proceed with some plan, the understanding gained from seminars will reduce the amount of time required of a lawyer to put a plan in place.

Seminar lawyers sometimes criticize local lawyers as inept and vice versa. A medical physicist should take the time required to understand fully the mechanisms of asset protection before deciding on a plan. A year of thinking about asset protection plans is not too long.

§ 43   What Attitude Is Appropriate

There is old wisdom that one does not sue one's friends or people one likes and respects. Though this saying may not be completely accurate, there is reason to believe that it is largely true. All health care delivery systems should strive to secure employees and health care professionals who not only provide quality technical service but also relate to patients in a positive, understanding, and supportive manner. This responsibility regarding attitude cannot be completely delegated; the chief or lead physicist should also exhibit these characteristics. People in an organization emulate the person in charge.

Everyone occasionally must make a decision that cannot satisfy all the competing interests. It may be as simple a question of where to allocate a limited amount of time. The authors suggest that the welfare of patients should come first, the welfare of the employing institution should come second, and the welfare of self or coworkers last. If the enterprise is successful, the individuals participating are also successful.

It is difficult for a medical physicist who becomes a defendant to see anything favorable resulting from a lawsuit. Yet an argument can be made that the possibility of a lawsuit, in some way or to some extent, serves to discipline a profession and to ensure the commitment of resources for sound physics and quality assurance. A further point can be made. The appearance in the legal arena of medical physicists or hospitals because of inadequate physics support may be, over time, one of the strongest forces for improvement of the general professional position of medical physicists.

EPILOGUE

§ 44 A Medical Physicist Encounters the Law (4) (Story continued from § 35)

In the trial the plaintiff, the plaintiff's expert witnesses, the defendants, and the defendant's expert witnesses testified. The plaintiff's attorney pointed out weaknesses in the statements of the defense witnesses, such as the uncertainty in the dose to the eye structures introduced by the loss of the eyeshield used for the plaintiff's treatment. He stated that the standard of care required certainty in the amount of dose delivered, that the standard of care was breached, and that the resulting overdose to structures under the eyeshield lead to injuries and serious damage to the plaintiff. Also he called attention to some discrepancies between the pretrial depositions and the trial testimony of witnesses.

The defense attorney raised a question about the seriousness of damage to the plaintiff's eye. The main complaint by the plaintiff was the loss of lubricating tear fluid in the affected eye. The plaintiff wore an eye patch throughout the trial. The defense attorney asked the plaintiff for his driver's license. This license had been renewed since the radiation treatments but did not show an eye patch in the plaintiff's picture. In testimony the plaintiff stated that he sometimes drove on long cross-country automobile trips. The defense attorney made the point that the electron-beam treatment was the best choice in this case. Surgery would have left the plaintiff without an eyelid or at least a highly distorted eyelid. Low-energy x-ray treatment posed the danger of permanent damage to the bone under the eyebrow. The defense attorney pointed out that the relatively minor eye complications experienced by the patient had been consented to by the plaintiff prior to treatment. Also, the patient may have contributed to these minor complications, in whole or in part, by his self-prescribed treatments of the eye with corticosteroids after completion of the radiation treatments. The defense attorney in his closing arguments stated that the plaintiff failed to prove breach of the standard of care and failed to show unexpected and unconsented to injury and damages—elements necessary to prove negligence on the part to the defendants.

After deliberating for four hours the jury returned. Both sides awaited the verdict expectantly.

The End

This story is based upon two real trials. Both of the trials resulted in a verdict and judgment in favor of the defendants. The plaintiffs took nothing. The story here is simple, but pretrial preparation and trial are complex and produce much paperwork. Each trial required about two weeks in court. In each case over five years elapsed from the time of the treatment to the time of the trial.

A well-known truism among lawyers holds that no one can be sure how a jury trial will turn out. All would agree that completeness of preparation and clarity in telling a comprehensible story on the part of parties, witnesses, and particularly the lawyers are of great importance.

REFERENCES

1 W. Keeton, ed., Prosser and Keeton on The Law of Torts, § 1 at 2, 6, 5th ed. 1984, West Publishing Co., St. Paul (with permission of the West Publishing Corporation).

2 W. Keeton, ed., Prosser and Keeton on the Law of Torts, § 75 at 534, 5th ed. 1984, West Publishing Co., St. Paul. This quote is a comment based on the writings of Oliver Wendell Holmes. O. Holmes, The Common Law, at 1, 2, (1881), Little, Brown and Co., Boston.

3 P. Huber, Liability: The Legal Revolution and Its Consequences, (1988), Basic Books, New York.

4 R. Neely, The Product Liability Mess: How Business Can Be Rescued from the Politics of State Courts, (1988) at 2 (1988), Free Press, New York.

5 MacKay v. St. Charles Medical Center, 804 P.2d 1192 at 1194 (Or. App. 1991).

6 Breast Cancer Ranks High for Malpractice Claims, American College of Radiology Bulletin, 8-95, at 26, (1995).

7 B. Franklin, Learning Curve, American Bar Association Journal, *81*, 62 at 65, (August, 1995).

8 American Medical Association, Special Task Force on Professional Liability and Insurance, Professional Liability in the 80's, Report 2, at 13, November (1984).

9 M. Middleton, A Changing Landscape. American Bar Association Journal, *81*, 56 at 59, (August, 1995).

10   W. Keeton, ed., Prosser and Keeton on the Law of Torts, § 30 at 164, 165, 5th ed. 1984, West Publishing Co., St. Paul (with permission of the West Publishing Corporation).

11   J. Perdue, The Law of Texas Medical Malpractice §7.03 at 257, (2d ed. 1985), 22 Hous. L. Rev. 1.

12   W. Keeton, ed., Prosser and Keeton on the Law of Torts, § 32 at 185, 5th ed. 1984, West Publishing Co., St. Paul.

13   W. Trail and S. Kelly-Claybrook, Health Care Providers, in J. Edgar, Jr. and J. Sales, Editorial Consultants, Texas Torts and Remedies § 11.01 [2] [b] at 17, (1989 with supp. to 1996), Mathew Bender and Co., Inc., New York.

14   W. Keeton, ed., Prosser and Keeton on The Law of Torts, § 37 at 238, 5th ed. 1984, West Publishing Co., St. Paul (with permission of the West Publishing Corporation).

15   W. Keeton, ed., Prosser and Keeton on the Law of Torts, § 32 at 187, 5th ed. 1984, West Publishing Co., St. Paul.

16   J. Perdue, The Law of Texas Malpractice, § 7.03 at 265, 22 Hous. L. Rev. 1, (2nd ed. 1985).

17   Helling v. Carey, 83 Wn 2d 514, 519 P2d 981 (Wn. 1974).

18   Helling v. Carey, 519 P.2d 981 at 986 (Wn. 1974).

19   Public Law 102-539 (106 Stat. 3547). Mammography Quality Standards Act of 1992. H.R. 6182 Washington, D.C.: House of Representatives, October 27, 1992.

20   W. Keeton, ed., Prosser and Keeton on the Law of Torts, § 36 at 233, 5th ed. 1984, West Publishing Co., St. Paul. See also, Restatement (Second) of Torts, §§ 285, 286, 288C (1965) American Law Institute Publisher, St. Paul (with permission of the West Publishing Corporation).

21   O'Conner v. Commonwealth Edison Col, 485 F. Supp. 566 at 567 (W.D. Okla. 1979).

22   Silkwood v. Kerr-McGee Corp., 748 F. Supp. 672 at 676 (C.D. Ill. 1990).

23   Hernandez v. Nueces County Medical Soc., 779 S.W. 2d 867 (Tex. App. 1989).

24   Hernandez v. Nueces County Medical Soc., 779 S.W. 2d 867 at 871 (Tex. App. 1989).

25   J. King, Jr., The Law of Medical Malpractice, ch. 5 at 201, (2nd ed. 1986), West Publishing Co., St. Paul.

26   W. Keeton, ed., Prosser and Keeton on the Law of Torts, § 42 at 272, 273, 5th ed. 1984, West Publishing Co., St. Paul (with permission of the West Publishing Corporation).

27   W. Keeton, ed., Prosser and Keeton on the Law of Torts, § 42 at 279, 5th ed. 1984, West Publishing Co., St. Paul (with permission of the West Publishing Corporation).

28 NCRP Statement No. 7, The Probability That a Particular Malignancy May Have Been Caused by a Specified Irradiation, September 30, 1992, National Council on Radiation Protection and Measurements, Bethesda.

29 D. Gooden, Proof of Facts, Radiation Injuries–Ionizing Radiation, § 14 at 119, (1991), Lawyers Cooperative Publishing, New York (available from Medical Physics Publishing, Madison).

30 NCRP Report No. 116, Limitation of Exposure to Ionizing Radiation, (1993), National Council on Radiation Protection and Measurements, Bethesda.

31 W. Sinclair, Radiation Protection: Recent Recommendations of the ICRP and the NCRP and Their Biological Basis, Advances in Radiation Biology *16*, 303, (1992), Academic Press, New York.

32 BEIR V, Health Effects of Exposure to Low Levels of Ionizing Radiation, Committee on the Biological Effects of Ionizing Radiation, (1990), National Academy Press, Washington.

33 Breast Cancer Study, at 4, June 1995, Physician Insurers Association of America, Washington.

34 W. Keeton, ed., Prosser and Keeton on the Law of Torts, §30 at 165, 5th ed. 1984, West Publishing Co., St. Paul.

35 Texas Civil Practice and Remedies Code, § 33.001; amended by Acts 1995, 74th Leg., ch. 136, § 1.

36 Texas Civil Practice and Remedies Code, § 33.012(a); amended by Acts 1995, 74th Leg., ch. 136, § 1.

37 E. Reynolds III, General Principles of Professional Liability, in J. Edgar, Jr. and J. Sales, Editorial Consultants, Texas Torts and Remedies, § 10.05 [7] at 34, (1989 with supp. to 1996), Mathew Bender and Co., Inc.

38 W. Trail and S. Kelley-Claybrook, Health Care Providers, in J. Edgar, Jr. and J. Sales, Editorial Consultants, Texas Torts and Remedies § 11.04 [1] at 67, (1989 with supp. to 1996), Mathew Bender and Co., Inc., New York.

39 W. Keeton, ed., Prosser and Keeton on The Law of Torts, § 34 at 212, 5th ed. 1984, West Publishing Co., St. Paul (with permission of the West Publishing Corporation).

40 E. Reynolds III, General Principles of Professional Liability, in J. Edgar, Jr. and J. Sales, Editorial Consultants, Texas Torts and Remedies, § 10.03 [2] [b] at 11, (1989 with supp. to 1996), Mathew Bender and Co., Inc., New York.

41 Transportation Ins. Co. v. Moriel, 879 S.W. 2d 10 at 23 (Tex. 1994).

42 Texas Civil Practice and Remedies Code, §§ 41.001 (7) (B), 41.003 (a)(2), and 41.003 (b); amended by Acts 1995, 74th Leg., ch. 19, § 1.

43 Texas Civil Practice and Remedies Code, § 41.008 (b); amended by Acts 1995, 74th Leg., ch. 19, § 1.

44 W. Trail and S. Kelley-Claybrook, Health Care Providers, in J. Edgar, Jr. and J. Sales, Editorial Consultants, Texas Torts and Remedies § 11.01 [4] at 38.1, (1989 with supp. to 1996), Mathew Bender and Co., Inc., New York.

45 E. Reynolds III, General Principles of Professional Liability, in J. Edgar, Jr. and J. Sales, Editorial Consultants, Texas Torts and Remedies, § 10.03 [2] [c] at 11, (1989 with supp. to 1996), Mathew Bender and Co., Inc.

46 Brown v. Comerford, 781 P.2d 857 (Or. App. 1989).

47 Brown v. Comerford, 781 P.2d 857 at 858 (Or. App. 1989).

48 Restatement (Second) of Torts, § 402A (1965) American Law Institute Publishers, St. Paul.

49 V. Brannigan and R. Dayhoff, Liability for Personal Injuries Caused by Defective Medical Computer Programs, 7 Am. J. Law and Med. 123, (1981).

50 Dubin v. Michael Reese Hospital and Medical Center, 393 NE 2d 588 (Ill. App., 1979); 415 NE 2d 350 (Ill., 1980).

51 Dubin v. Michael Reese Hospital and Medical Center, 415 N.E. 2d 350 at 352 (Ill. 1980).

52 Nevauex v. Park Place Hospital, Inc. 656 S.W. 2d 923 at 926 (Tex. App. 1983).

53 B. Roswit and F. Bensel, Medical Liability in the Practice of Therapeutic Radiology. Int. J. Radiation Oncology Biol. Phys. 2, 553, (1977).

54 J. Perdue, The Law of Texas Medical Malpractice, § 1.02 at 10, (2nd ed. 1985), 22 Hous. L. Rev. 1.

55 Wynn v. Mid-Cities Clinic, 628 S.W. 2d 809 at 812 (Tex. App. 1981)

56 State v. Kluttz, 175 S.E. 81 at 82 (N.C., 1934).

57 D. Becham, Federal Rules, Annotated, Texas Lawyer Press, Dallas, 1995.

58 Vernon's Texas Rules Annotated, Rules of Civil Evidence, 1995 Special Pamphlet, West Publishing Co., St Paul.

59 Texas Health and Safety Code §§ 161.031 and 161.032; Acts 1989, 71st Leg., ch. 678, § 1.

60 W. Trail and S. Kelley-Claybrook, Health Care Providers, in J. Edgar, Jr. and J. Sales, Editorial Consultants, Texas Torts and Remedies § 11.05 [3] [d] at 99, (1989 with supp. to 1996), Mathew Bender and Co., Inc., New York.

61 F. James, Jr. and G. Hazard, Jr., Civil Procedure, § 11.2 at 529, (2nd ed. 1977), Little, Brown and Co., Boston.

62 J. Perdue, The Law of Texas Malpractice, § 1.01 at 2, (2d ed. 1985), 22 Hous L. Rev.1.

63 Baird v. Sickler, 433 N. E. 2d 593 at 595, (Ohio, 1982).

64 J. King, Jr., The Laws of Medical Malpractice, Ch 6 at 239, (2d ed. 1986), West Publishing Co., St. Paul.

65 J. Perdue, The Law of Texas Malpractice, § 4 at 143 and § 5 at 175, (2nd ed. 1985), 22 Hous. L. Rev. 1.

66 J. King, Jr., The Law of Medical Malpractice, Ch 9 at 298, (2d ed. 1986), West Publishing Co., St. Paul.

67 W. Trail and S. Kelly-Claybrook, Health Care Providers, § 11.02 at 52.2 in J. Edgar, Jr. and J. Sales, Editorial Consultants, Texas Torts and Remedies, (1989 with supp. to 1996), Mathew Bender, New York.

68 W. Keeton, ed., Prosser and Keeton on the Law of Torts, § 54 at 359, 5th ed. 1984, West Publishing Co., St. Paul (with permission of the West Publishing Corporation).

69 W. Menges, The Negligent Nurse: Rx for the Medical Malpractice Victim. 12 Tulsa L.J. 104 at 105, (1976).

70 Baur v. Mesta Machine Co., 176 A. 2d 684 at 688 (Pa. 1961).

71 Lunsford v. Board of Nurse Examiners, 648 S.W. 2d 391 at 394, 395 (Tex. App. 1983).

72 Dougherty v. Gifford, 826 S. W. 2d 668 at 674 (Tex. App. 1992).

73 Stevenson v. Golden, 276 N. W. 849 at 857 (Mich. 1937).

74 Marion Malleable Iron Works v. Baldwin, 145 N.E. 559 at 560 (Ind. App. 1924).

75 Corletto v. Shore Memorial Hospital, 350A.2d 534 at 537 (N.J. Super. 1975).

76 Purcell v. Zimbelman, 500 P.2d 335 at 343 (Ariz. App. 1972).

77 J. Perdue, The Law of Texas Malpractice, § 5.04 at 199, (2d ed. 1985), 22 Hous. L. Rev. 1.

78 American Association of Physicists in Medicine, Report No. 33, Staffing Levels and Responsibilities of Physicists in Diagnostic Radiology, § III A2 at 7, (1991), American Institute of Physics, Woodbury, NY.

79 American Association of Physicists in Medicine, Report No. 42, The Role of the Clinical Medical Physicist in Diagnostic Radiology at 14, 15, (1994), American Institute of Physics, Woodbury, NY.

80 American Association of Physicists in Medicine, Report No. 38, Statement on the Role of a Physicist in Radiation Oncology, at 8, 9, (1993), American Institute of Physics, Woodbury, NY.

81 American Association of Physicists in Medicine, Report of AAPM Radiation Therapy Task Group 40 (also called AAPM Report No. 46), Comprehensive QA for Radiation Oncology, Med. Phys. *21*, 581 at 586, (1994).

82 Joint Commission on the Accreditation of Healthcare Organizations: Radiation Oncology Services, Quality Assurance Standards, (1987).

83 Joint Commission on the Accreditation of Healthcare Organizations: Radiation Oncology Services, Quality Assurance Standards, (1992).

84 American Association of Physicists in Medicine, Report of AAPM Radiation Therapy Task Group 40 (also called AAPM Report No.

46), Comprehensive QA for Radiation Oncology, Med. Phys. *21*, 581 at 584, (1994).

85   American Association of Physicists in Medicine, Report of AAPM Radiation Therapy Task Group 40 (also called AAPM Report No. 46), Comprehensive QA for Radiation Oncology, Med. Phys. *21*, 581 at 587, (1994).

86   W. Menges, Jr., The Negligent Nurse: Rx for the Medical Malpractice Victim, 12 Tulsa L.R., 104 at 117, (1976).

87   D. Brushwood, Medical Malpractice Pharmacy Law, § 4.07 at 41, 42, (1986), McGraw-Hill Book Co., New York.

88   Norton v. Argonaut Insurance Co., 144 So. 2d 249 at 260, (La. App. 1962).

89   R. Steeves and F. Patterson, Legal Responsibility of the Hospital Pharmacist for Rational Drug Therapy, American Journal of Hospital Pharmacy, *26*, 404 at 406 (1969).

90   Lunsford v. Board of Nurse Examiners, 648 S.W. 2d 391 at 394 (Tex. App., 1983).

91   American Association of Physicists in Medicine, Report No. 42, The Role of the Clinical Medical Physicist in Diagnostic Radiology at 14, (1994), American Institute of Physics, Woodbury, NY.

92   M. Rozenfield and D. Jette, Quality Assurance of Radiation Dosage: Usefulness of Redundancy. Radiology, *150*, 241, (1984).

93   American Association of Physicists in Medicine, The Roles, Responsibilities and Status of the Clinical Medical Physicists, (1986), American Institute of Physics, Woodbury, NY.

94   American Association of Physicists in Medicine, Report No. 38 at 8, The Role of the Physicist in Radiation Oncology, (1993), American Institute of Physics, Woodbury, NY.

95   American Association of Physicist in Medicine, Report of AAPM Radiation Therapy Task Group 40 (also called AAPM Report No. 46), Comprehensive QA for Radiation Oncology, Med. Phys. *21*, 581 at 612, (1994).

96   American Association of Physicists in Medicine, Report No. 42 at 13, The Role of the Clinical Medical Physicist in Diagnostic Radiology, (1994),. American Institute of Physics, Woodbury, NY.

97   National Council on Radiation Protection and Measurements, Limitation of Exposure to Ionizing Radiation. NCRP Report No. 116 at 37, (1993), Bethesda.

98   Committee on the Biological Effects of Ionizing Radiation, Health Effects of Exposure to Low Levels of Ionizing Radiation, BEIR V, Ch. 6 at 352, (1990), National Academy Press, Washington.

99   R. Brent, Radiation Teratogenesis: Fetal Risk and Abortion, Biological Risks of Medical Irradiations, G. Fullerton, D. Kopp, R. Waggener, and E. Webster eds. at 223, (1980), American Associa-

REFERENCES 95

tion of Physicists in Medicine, American Institute of Physics, Woodbury, NY.

100 E. Hall, Radiobiology for the Radiologist, Ch. 20 at 399, (2nd ed. 1978), Harper and Row, Hagerstown, MD.

101 American Association of Physicists in Medicine, Report of AAPM Radiation Therapy Task Group #36 (also called AAPM Report No. 50), Fetal Dose from Radiotherapy with Photon Beams, Med. Phys. 22, 63, (1995).

102 American Association of Physicists in Medicine, Report of AAPM Radiation Therapy Task Group #34 (also called AAPM Report No. 45), Management of Radiation Oncology Patients with Implanted Cardiac Pacemakers, Med. Phys. 21, 85, (1994).

103 National Council on Radiation Protection and Measurements, Report No. 69, Dosimetry of X-Ray and Gamma Ray Beams for Radiation Therapy in the Energy Range 10 keV to 50 MeV § 6.6 at 69, (1981), Bethesda.

104 American Association of Physicists in Medicine, Symposium Proceedings No. 3, Proceedings of a Symposium on Quality Assurance of Radiotherapy Equipment, G. Starkschall, ed., (1982), American Institute of Physics, Woodbury, NY.

105 American Association of Physicists in Medicine, Report No. 13, Physical Aspects of Quality Assurance in Radiation Therapy, (1984), American Institute of Physics, Woodbury, NY.

106 American College of Medical Physics, Report No. 2, Radiation Control and Quality Assurance in Radiation Oncology, A Suggested Protocol, (1986), Reston, VA.

107 American Association of Physicists in Medicine, Report No. 24, Radiotherapy Portal Imaging Quality, American Institute of Physics, (1987), Woodbury, NY.

108 American College of Medical Physics Symposium, Quality Assurance in Radiotherapy Physics, G. Starkschall and J. Horton, eds., (1991), Medical Physics Publishing, Madison.

109 American Association of Physicists in Medicine, Comprehensive QA for Radiation Oncology, Report of AAPM Radiation Therapy Committee Task Group 40 (also called AAPM Report no. 46), Med. Phys. 21, 581, (1994).

110 American Association of Physicists in Medicine, AAPM Code of Practice for Radiotherapy Accelerators Report of AAPM Radiation Therapy Task Group #45 (also called AAPM Report 47), Med. Phys. 21, 1093, (1994).

111 American Association of Physicists in Medicine, Report No. 55, Radiation Treatment Planning Dosimetry Verification, (1995), AAPM, College Park, MD.

112   National Council on Radiation Protection and Measurements, Report No. 30, Safe Handling of Radioactive Materials, (1964), Bethesda.
113   American Association of Physicists in Medicine, Report No. 6, Scintillation Camera Acceptance Testing and Performance Evaluation, (1980), American Institute of Physics, Woodbury, NY.
114   American Association of Physicists in Medicine, Report No. 9, Computer-Aided Scintillation Camera Acceptance Testing, (1981), American Institute of Physics, Woodbury, NY.
115   National Council on Radiation Protection and Measurements, Report No. 58, A Handbook of Radioactivity Measurements Procedures, (2nd ed. 1985), Bethesda.
116   American College of Medical Physics, Report No. 3, Radiation Control and Quality Assurance Surveys-Nuclear Medicine: A Suggested Protocol, (1986), Reston, VA.
117   American Association of Physicists in Medicine, Report No. 22, Rotation Scintillation Camera Spect Acceptance Testing and Quality Control, (1987), American Institute of Physics, Woodbury, NY.
118   American Association of Physicists in Medicine, Quantification of SPECT Performance, Report of AAPM Nuclear Medicine Committee Task Group #4 (also called AAPM Report No. 52), Med. Phys. *22*, 401, (1995).
119   W. Hendee, and R. Rossi, Quality Assurance for Radiographic X-Ray Units and Associated Equipment, HEW Publication (FDA) 79-8094, U.S. Department of Health, Education and Welfare (1979), Rockville, MD.
120   American Association of Physicists in Medicine, Report No. 8, Pulse Echo Ultrasound Imaging Systems: Performance Tests and Criteria, (1980), American Institute of Physics, Woodbury, NY.
121   American College of Radiology, Mammography Quality Control, Committee on Quality Assurance in Mammography (1992).
122   American Association of Physicists in Medicine, Report #15, Performance Evaluation and Quality Assurance in Digital Subtraction Angiography, (1985), American Institute of Physics. Woodbury, NY.
123   American College of Medical Physics, Report No. 1, Radiation Control and Quality Assurance Surveys-Diagnostic Radiology, A Suggested Protocol, (1986), Reston, VA
124   National Council on Radiation Protection and Measurements, NCRP Report No. 99, Quality Assurance for Diagnostic Imaging Equipment, (1988), Bethesda.
125   American Association of Physicists in Medicine, Report No. 29, Equipment Requirement and Quality Control for Mammography, (1990), American Institute of Physics, Woodbury, NY.

126 American Association of Physicists in Medicine, Report No. 31, Standardized Methods for Measuring Diagnostic X-ray Exposures, (1990), American Institute of Physics, Woodbury, NY.

127 American Association of Physicists in Medicine, Report No. 39, Specification and Acceptance Testing of Computed Tomography Scanners, (1993), American Institute of Physics, Woodbury, NY.

128 American Association of Physicists in Medicine, Summer School 1991, Specification, Acceptance Testing and Quality Control of Diagnostic X-Ray Imaging Equipment, J. Seibert, G. Barnes, R. Gould, eds. American Association of Physicists in Medicine, Monograph No. 20, (1994), American Institute of Physics, Woodbury, NY.

129 L. Cohen, T. Schultheiss, and R. Kennaugh, A Radiation Overdose Incident: Initial Data. Int. J. Radiat. Oncol. Biol. Phys. *33*, 217, (1995).

130 W. Gagnon, P. Kennedy, L. Berkley, W. Hanson, and R. Shalek, An Analysis of Discrepancies Encountered by the AAMP Radiological Physics Center, Med. Phys. *5*, 556, (1978).

131 L. Berkley, W. Hanson, and R. Shalek, Discussion of the Characteristics and Results of Measurements with a Portable Well Ionization Chamber for Calibration of Brachytherapy Sources, Recent Advances in Brachytherapy Physics, D. Shearer, ed. AAPM Monograph #7, at 38, (1981).

132 Darling v. Charleston Community Memorial Hospital, 211 N.E. 2d 253 (Ill. 1965).

133 Cohen v. Citizens National Trust and Savings Bank, 300 P. 2d 14 at 16 (Cal. App. 1956).

134 W. Keeton, ed., Prosser and Keeton on the Law of Torts § 106 at 738, 5th ed. 1984, West Publishing Co., St. Paul (with permission of the West Publishing Corporation).

135 W. Keeton, ed., Prosser and Keeton on the Law of Torts § 106 at 739, 5th ed. 1984, West Publishing Co., St. Paul (with permission of the West Publishing Corporation).

136 Medical Use of Byproduct Material, 10CFR (1-1-94 Edition) Part 35 §§ 35.2, 35.32, 35.33.

137 R. Shalek, A Case for Some Deregulation in Radiation Therapy, Current Regulatory Issues in Medical Physics, M. Martin and J. Smathers, ed. 147 at 149, (1992),. American College of Medical Physics, Reston, VA.

138 The National Foundation for Asset Protection and Estate Preservation, 1675 North Freedom Blvd. #5-B, Provo, UT 84604.

GLOSSARY

AAPM   American Association of Physicists in Medicine.

ACTOR   The doer. One who acts.

ADMISSIBLE EVIDENCE   Evidence which may be received by a trial court to aid the trier of fact (the jury or judge in a non-jury trial).

AGENT   One authorized to act for another party called the principal.

ALTERNATIVE DISPUTE RESOLUTION (ADR)   Methods of resolving disputes outside of court such as mediation or arbitration.

APPARENT AGENT (OSTENSIBLE AGENT)   One who is not an agent of a principal but because of the actions or omissions of the principal was reasonably relied upon as an agent by a third person to that person's detriment.

APPEAL   The complaint to a superior court of error committed by an inferior court.

APPELLATE COURT   A court available for review of the rulings and judgments of a trial court.

ARBITRATION   The submission of a dispute for determination to private unofficial persons. Usually the decision is binding upon the parties and has the force of a court decision.

BORROWED SERVANT   An employee of one person or entity (such as a hospital) placed under the control and direction of another (such as a physician).

BREACH OF DUTY   A failure to perform a duty owed to another.

BURDEN OF GOING FORWARD WITH THE EVIDENCE   Responsibility of presenting evidence in support of a given proposition.

BURDEN OF PERSUASION   Responsibility of establishing a pleading by plaintiff against all counterarguments.

BURDEN OF PROOF   Burden of persuasion and the burden of going forward with the evidence.

CAPTAIN OF THE SHIP   A doctrine that holds the physician in charge (particularly a surgeon) responsible for whatever occurs. This doctrine is not of great importance in 1996.

CAUSATION IN FACT   The defendant's action or omission caused the harm to the plaintiff.

CHALLENGE (A juror)   Rejection of a juror for cause such as relationship of a juror to a party; each side may reject a fixed number of jurors without cause.

CLEAR AND CONVINCING   Standard of proof greater than preponderance of the evidence (usual civil standard) but less than beyond a reasonable doubt (criminal standard).

COMMON LAW   Legal system based on judicial precedent rather than legislative enactments.

COMPENSATORY DAMAGES   Damages that will compensate the injured party for the injuries sustained and nothing more. Also called actual damages.

CONTINGENCY FEE   An attorney's charge based upon a successful outcome of a lawsuit. It is usually an agreed percentage of the plaintiff's recovery of damages.

CONTRACTOR OR INDEPENDENT CONTRACTOR   One who makes an agreement with another to do a piece of work, retaining in himself or herself control of the means, method and manner of producing the result.

CONTRIBUTORY NEGLIGENCE   Lack of care on part of plaintiff that concurring with the negligence of defendant is the proximate cause of the injury to the plaintiff. Same as proportionate responsibility.

THE COURT   The judge, or body of judges, presiding over a court. The court decides matters of law and if there is no jury also matters of fact.

CRIME   A wrong determined by the government to be injurious to the common good and to be prosecutable.

CROSS-EXAMINATION   Questioning by an opposing party on evidence offered by a witness.

DAMAGES   Monetary compensation awarded to a party injured by another.

DECEIT   A false representation of a fact made with knowledge of its falsity or made recklessly upon which another relies to his detriment or injury.

DEFAULT JUDGMENT   Judgment rendered as a consequence of the non-appearance of the defendant.

DEFENDANT   The party responding to the complaint of a plaintiff.

DEFENDANT'S PLEADING   Statements in legal form in answer to a plaintiff's pleading constituting the grounds of defense.

DEPOSITION   Method of pretrial discovery involving questions and answers of a witness under oath with cross-examination.

DIRECT CORPORATE LIABILITY   Liability based on the direct, non-delegable duty a hospital owes to its patients.

DIRECTED VERDICT   Verdict returned by the jury at the direction of the trial judge in favor of a party if the opposing party fails to present a requisite minimum of evidence.

DISCOVERY   Disclosure of facts and documents known or held by the adverse party.

DUTY   Obligatory conduct owed by one person to another.

EVIDENCE   Means by which alleged matter of fact is proved or disproved.

EXEMPLARY DAMAGES   Compensation in excess of actual damages as enhancement to the injured plaintiff, or as punishment to the defendant and deterrent of future similar actions by the defendant or others.

EXPERT WITNESS   One with skilled experience or extensive knowledge relevant to issues being adjudicated and who may draw conclusions from facts.

FORESEEABILITY   Reasonable anticipation of harm or injury likely to result from acts or failure to act.

GROSS NEGLIGENCE   Action involving an extreme degree of risk to others of which the actor is aware yet proceeds in conscious indifference to the rights, safety, or welfare of others.

HEARSAY   Second hand evidence that depends for its creditability on someone other than the witness. Hearsay evidence is not admitted in court except under a hearsay exception.

HEARSAY EXCEPTION   Hearsay that under certain circumstances is admitted into evidence.

IMPEACHING A WITNESS   Providing evidence that the testimony of a witness is unworthy of credibility.

INDEMNIFICATION   Generally, compensation for loss   Where liability of a person arises through the action of law (e.g. liability of an employer) that person can seek indemnification against the negligent actor.

INJURY   Damage to another's person, right, or property—a violation of a legal right.

INTENTIONAL TORTS   Implies purpose or intent to injure.

INTERLOCUTORY   Provisional, not final.

INTERROGATORIES   Pretrial discovery tool in which written questions are served on the adverse party who must give written replies under oath.

JOINDER   Uniting two or more elements into one.

JOINT AND SEVERAL LIABILITY   If defendants are jointly and severally liable all or any one of the defendants may be sued for full satisfaction of damages.

JOINT REPRESENTATION   Two or more parties represented by the same attorney.

JUDGE   Presiding officer of a court; rules on questions of law.

JUDGMENT   A determination of the rights of parties by the judge.

JUDGMENT NOTWITHSTANDING THE VERDICT   Judgment (by judge) reversing a jury verdict that had no reasonable support in fact or was contrary to law.

JUDGMENT ON THE VERDICT   Judgment for the party obtaining the verdict.

JURY A certain number of persons, selected according to law, sworn to inquire into matters of fact and declare the truth based on evidence laid before them.

LACK OF CAPACITY In this context, not having the right to sue.

LAWYER-CLIENT PRIVILEGE Communications between a client and a lawyer that need not be disclosed.

LEGISLATURE Assembly of persons that make laws for states or the nation.

LIABILITY An obligation or responsibility to do or refrain from doing something.

LIABILITY INSURANCE Indemnity against liability.

LIMITED PARTNERSHIP A partnership managed by a general partner who has unlimited liability and having limited partners who do not participate in management but have liability limited to their capital contributed.

LITIGANT A party involved in a lawsuit.

LITIGATION A controversy in court in which the plaintiff seeks to enforce a legal right.

LOST CHANCE DUE TO DELAYED DIAGNOSIS Delay in diagnosis resulting in decreased probability of successful treatment.

MALPRACTICE Any professional misconduct.

MATERIAL Related and necessary to an issue in question.

MEDIATION Intervention of a third person to reconcile contending parties Negotiations are not binding upon either party.

MISADMINISTRATION In this context a delivery of radiation or radioactivity to a patient differing in quantity from that intended and exceeding a limit set by governmental regulations. A report to a regulatory agency is required.

MQSA Mammography Quality Standards Act.

NCRP National Council on Radiation Protection and Measurements.

NEGLIGENCE Failure to exercise that degree of care a person of ordinary prudence (a reasonable man) would exercise under the same circumstances. A tort having the elements of duty, breach of duty, causation of injury, and damages.

NON-ECONOMIC DAMAGES   Damages that cannot be estimated and compensated by money, e.g., disfigurement.

NOTIFICATION OF DEFECT   Information relating to a defect in a product sent by a manufacturer to an owner of the equipment.

OATH   Affirmation of the truth of testimony by a witness. If the testimony is proved to be false the witness may be criminally prosecuted for perjury.

PARTY   Plaintiff or defendant.

PECUNIARY LOSS   Loss of money or a loss that can be calculated in money.

PEER PRIVILEGE   Defined here to mean that records and proceedings of a hospital or medical organization committee are confidential and not subject to court subpoena.

PERJURY   Criminal offense of making false statements under oath.

PETITION   A formal written request for a certain thing to be done.

PHYSICIAN-PATIENT RELATIONSHIP   A voluntary, contractual relationship between a physician and a patient, created by an expressed or implied agreement.

PLAINTIFF   One who brings a lawsuit.

PLAINTIFF'S PLEADING   Written statements in legal form which constitutes the plaintiff's cause of action.

PREPONDERANCE OF THE EVIDENCE   Proof that leads the trier of fact (jury or judge in a non-jury trial) to find the existence of a fact in issue more probable than not.

PRINCIPAL   One who gives authority to an agent to act for him or her.

PRIVILEGED COMMUNICATION   Permitted resistance of legal pressure to disclose the contents of a communication, e.g. lawyer-client communication.

PRIVITY   In this context, the relationship existing between contracting parties.

PROCEDURE   Mode of proceeding by which a legal right is enforced.

PRODUCTION OF TANGIBLE THINGS   An enforceable pretrial discovery procedure for obtaining documents and other things from the other party for copying or photographing.

PRODUCTS LIABILITY A manufacturer or seller is held to be strictly liable for injuries caused by defect in his product without a showing of fault.

PROPORTIONATE RESPONSIBILITY Same as contributory negligence.

PROXIMATE CAUSE The dominant or legal cause of an injury without which cause the injury would not have occurred.

PUNITIVE DAMAGES Damages awarded as punishment. Included in the term exemplary damages.

QUALITY ASSURANCE PRINCIPLES General recommendations, as opposed to QA Guidelines relating to particular equipment or procedures.

"REASONABLE MAN" STANDARD A hypothetical person who exercises those qualities which society requires of its members for the protection of their own interest and the interests of others.

REASONABLE MEDICAL PROBABILITY OR REASONABLE MEDICAL CERTAINTY More probable than not, not mere conjecture, that event A caused event B or will cause event C.

RECORDABLE EVENT In this context, a delivery of radiation or radioactivity to a patient differing in quantity from that intended and exceeding a limit set by governmental regulations. The difference is smaller than that in a misadministration. A record is kept but no report to the regulatory agency is required.

RECORDED RECOLLECTION A record made at the time of the occurrence concerning a matter about which a witness once had personal knowledge but now has insufficient recollection to testify fully without referral to the record.

RELEVANT EVIDENCE Evidence having a tendency to make the existence of a fact more or less probable.

REQUEST FOR ADMISSIONS Pretrial discovery device by which one party asks another for affirmation of a fact or issue in order to reduce the number of issues to be litigated.

RES JUDICATA A thing decided; a settled legal issue.

RESPONDEAT SUPERIOR Let the superior reply.

REMITTUR Any reduction in damages by the court without consent of the jury. Party adversely affected can accept the reduced amount or have a new trial.

RSO   Radiation Safety Officer.

STANDARD OF CARE   Defines the duty of one person to another in a given situation. Used frequently in medical situations.

STATUTE   An act of legislature enacted into law governing conduct within its scope.

STATUTE OF LIMITATIONS   A law that fixes the time within which a party must initiate judicial action.

STRICT LIABILITY   Liability without a showing of fault for certain activities.

SUBPOENA   An order of a court to compel the appearance of a witness at a judicial proceeding.

SUMMARY JUDGMENT   Judgment made by a judge prior to jury verdict if there is no dispute as to facts or if only a question of law is involved.

SUPPLEMENTAL PLEADING   Altered or amended pleadings of a plaintiff or defendant.

SUPREME COURT   A court of high powers and extensive jurisdiction, existing in most states. In the federal judicial system it is the court of last resort.

TESTIMONY   Evidence by a competent witness under oath; as distinguished from evidence in writings.

TOLLING THE STATUTE OF LIMITATIONS   To show facts that remove the bar of judicial action, i.e., to extend the time period in which judicial action may be taken.

TORT   A private or civil wrong independent of contract.

TRADE SECRETS   A formula or process, not patented, known only to owner and selected employees of a business.

VERDICT   The opinion of a jury, or a judge in a non-jury trial, on a question of fact that the trial court may accept or reject in formulating its judgment.

VICARIOUS LIABILITY   By law the placing of liability for the actions of one person on another (e.g., an employer may be responsible for the actions of an employee).

WITNESS   A general witness is one who testifies to what he has seen, heard of otherwise observed. A plaintiff or defendant may be a witness.

WORK PRODUCT   Work done by attorney for a client (e.g., notes) that is ordinarily not subject to discovery.

ABOUT THE AUTHORS

ROBERT SHALEK had a 37 year career in Medical Physics at the University of Texas M. D. Anderson Cancer Center in Houston, serving 24 years as Chairman of the Physics Department. He was involved principally with radiation therapy but also had responsibilities in nuclear medicine, diagnostic radiology, and radiation protection.

He was born in 1922 and as a child lived in Oak Park, Illinois. His education consisted of a Bachelor's Degree in Physics from the University of Illinois, a Master's Degree in Mathematics from Southern Methodist University and a Master's Degree in Physics and Ph.D. in Biophysics from Rice University. A postdoctoral year followed at the Royal Cancer Hospital (now Royal Marsden) in London. Late in life a law degree from the University of Houston (evenings) provided to him the basis for passing the Texas Bar Examination and obtaining credentials to practice law in Texas. Early on, the educational progression was interrupted by $3\frac{1}{2}$ years in the U.S. Army and almost a year working on a geophysics (petroleum) crew. He married Elaine Chudleigh in 1951 and they have six grown children.

In retirement he has returned to working out-of-doors with a start-up independent oil company. While the oil patch claims priority, there has been time for him to work on several medical-legal cases a year as an expert, to give half a dozen lectures a year on subjects in this book, and to work on a few writing projects.

DAVID GOODEN is the Director of Biomedical Physics at Saint Francis Hospital in Tulsa. For almost 27 years he has served Saint Francis Hospital as radiation safety officer and radiological physicist for diagnostic x-ray, radiation therapy and nuclear medicine. Dr. Gooden is

Chairman of the Radiation Management Advisory Council for Oklahoma's Department of Environmental Quality. He has B.S. and M.S. degrees in physics from Emory University in Atlanta, a Ph.D. in nuclear reactor engineering from the University of Missouri, and a J.D. from Tulsa University. Dr. Gooden has provided radiation safety consultation in many areas, including health care, veterinary medicine, nuclear reactors, electric utilities, universities, industrial radiography, waste management, scrap metal salvage, foundries, and oil and gas production. His published works include subjects in medical physics and the legal aspects of radiation injury. Dr. Gooden is certified by the American Board of Health Physics (health physics), the American Board of Radiology (radiological physics), and the American Board of Medical Physics (radiation oncology physics). Dr. Gooden's primary legal interests lie in the areas of medical physics, radiation protection regulation, and radiation injury, especially late injury.

INDEX